English / French Medical Dictionary

Français / Anglais Dictionnaire Médical

D1728648

by John C. Rigdon

English / French Medical Dictionary
Français / Anglais Dictionnaire Médical

By John C. Rigdon

1st Printing – August 2015 0/0/0/0/CS

Published by:
Eastern Digital Resources
31 Bramblewood Drive SW
Cartersville, GA 30120
http://www.krengle.net
EMAIL: sales@krengle.net
Tel. (678) 739-9177

Introduction

This book is intended to assist English speakers who are visiting West African countries where French is primarily used. It is not intended to be an exhaustive study of the French language, but serve as an introduction and overview.

The author is not proficient in French. While I have tried to be as accurate as possible, I'm sure you'll find errors in this edition. Please direct corrections, comments, suggestions to jrigdon@krengle.net.

Contents

Sources Used

http://www.krengle.net/translate/pmwiki.php?n=Burkina.Home

http://ielanguages.com/frenchphonetics.html

http://www.pronunciationguide.info/French.html

A Guide to French Pronunciation

French uses the same alphabet as English, so the first inclination would be to pronounce it that way, but as you well know, nothing can be further than the truth. French pronunciation has also influenced the native languages of Africa although in most cases the native languages predate French.

French, like English, is not written phonetically. Vowels can be represented by several different letter combinations and many letters are actually not pronounced. (You can thank early "linguists" who changed the spelling of many French words, with complete disregard to pronunciation, so that it was closer to Latin orthography.)

French takes a while to get the hang of, but there are two things in our favor:

1. Most people already have a good general idea of what it's supposed to sound like.
2. Many of the most peculiar features of French pronunciation were inherited by English, and are thus somewhat familiar to us.

The most difficult challenges are getting the vowels right, and knowing when *not* to pronounce certain letters.

Sorting It All Out

First the easy part. The consonants are all pronounced pretty much the same. There are subtle differences in some letters, but for our use you can treat them the same and finesse them as you become more proficient.

Consonants

If you really want to study the differences in consonants:

These are generally silent at ends of words, except for four particular consonants: *c, r, f* and *l* (the consonants in the word "careful"); one exception to this is the final *-er*, which is pronounced **ay**, as noted above. Consonants followed by a silent *e* are pronounced.

c [+a,o,u]	**k**
c [+i,e]	**s**
ce [+vowel]	**s**, e.g. *Morceau* = **mor-<u>soh</u>**
ç	**s**
Ch	**sh**
g [+a,o,u]	**g**, hard, as in "go"
g [+I,e]	**zh**, like the *s* in "measure"
ge [+vowel]	**zh**, e.g. *Georges* = **zhorzh**
Gn	**ny**, like Italian *gn* or Spanish *ñ*
gu [+i,e,y]	**g**, hard, e.g. *Guillaume* = **gee-<u>yohm</u>**

H	**silent**, e.g. *Le Havre* = **luh <u>ahv</u>-ruh**
J	**zh**, like the *s* in "measure"
Lh	**y**, e.g. *Milhaud* = **mee-<u>yoh</u>**
ll	**l** by default (e.g. *village* = **vee-<u>lahzh</u>**, *allez* = **ah-<u>lay</u>**), but if the letters *ill* appear between two more vowels, the *ll* means **y** (e.g. *Guillaume* = **gee-<u>yohm</u>**)
qu	**k**, almost always, but occasionally **kw**, e.g. *quatuor* = **<u>kwah</u>-tü-or**
r	**r**: uvular (light gutteral) trill, usually silent after e at ends of words
s (between vowels)	**z**, e.g. *désir* = **day-<u>zeer</u>**
s (otherwise)	**s**
ss	**s**
tch	**ch**, as in "church"
th	**t**, e.g. *Jean-Yves Thibaudet* = **zhahn-eev tee-boh-<u>day</u>**
ti [+vowel]	**sy**, e.g. *nation* = **nah-<u>syo</u>^{n}**
x (non-final)	**z**
x (final)	**silent**, or **ks** (when following *i*, e.g. *Astérix* = **ah-steh-<u>reeks</u>**), or *s* (e.g. *dix* = **dees**, the number "ten")

z	**z**

Stress

Almost always on the last syllable (there are always exceptions). *Stress is absolutely unaffected by accent marks!*

Those who speak French may tell you that this rule is an oversimplification, that in reality, there is no stress in French. This means simply that when French is spoken properly, the syllables in any sentence or phrase run together in a continuous unaccented stream until they reach the end, and the final syllable of the stream sounds stressed because it is followed by a pause. In practice, this way of looking at it usually leads to the same result; in any case one should try to produce a smooth flow of syllables when pronouncing French, and not to overaccentuate any words in the middle of a phrase.

Linking

Final consonants that would otherwise be silent are pronounced, if the next word is related and begins with a vowel or mute *h*. Such sequences should be pronounced as a single word (e.g. *beaux* = **boh**, but *Beaux Arts Trio* = **bohz-ar** "trio" (or **bohz-art**), *bon* = **bo^n**, but *bon ami* = **bo-nah-mee**).

Elision

Contractions are signified by apostrophes, as in English. If you see an apostrophe, pretend it isn't there and pronounce every letter you see accordingly, e.g. *D'un Soir Triste* = **du^n swahr treest**

Notable Exceptions

The following important names break one or more of the rules stated above, so you'll just have to memorize them:

Auber	**oh-<u>behr</u>**
Berlioz	**<u>behr</u>-lee-ohz**
Pierre Boulez	**pyehr boo-<u>lehz</u>**
Guillaume Dufay	**gee-yohm dü-<u>fiy</u>** (**iy** sounds like "eye")
Darius Milhaud	**dah-ree-üs mee-<u>yoh</u>**
Francis Poulenc	**fro^n-<u>sees</u> <u>poo</u>-lenk**

1. [p], [t] and [k] are NOT aspirated in French so try not to let that extra puff of air escape from your lips.

2. Consonants that are alveolar in English are generally dental in French. Try to rest your tongue just behind your teeth instead of on the alveolar ridge for [t], [d], [s], [z], [l] and [n].

3. The letter **h** is never pronounced, but you need to remember to distinguish the *h non-aspiré* from the *h aspiré*. Most words belong to the first group, but

for the words that have an h aspiré, there are two characteristics that make them different: the definite article does not reduce to l' (called elision) but remains le or la and word boundaries are maintained so that sounds do not link (absence of liaison - see below). Most words with an h aspiré are   of   Germanic   origin.

1. **[R]** is articulated further back in the throat (with the back of the tongue) and is usually the hardest French consonant for English speakers to pronounce correctly. It is a voiced uvular fricative sound and does not have an effect on preceding vowels the way that American English r does. It must remain consistent in all positions, regardless of the other vowels and consonants that may be adjacent to it.

Initial	After consonant	Intervocalic	Before consonant	Final
rusé	droit	arrêt	partout	mer
rang	gris	courir	merle	pire
rose	trou	pleurer	corde	sourd

2. In the majority of words with the grapheme **ch**, the pronunciation is **[ʃ]**, but it is also pronounced **[k]** in words of Greek origin. It is silent, however, in the word *almanach*.

ch = [ʃ]   ch = [k]

chercher   archéologie
réchauffer chaos
chérubin   chrétien
architecte écho
catéchisme orchestre
Achille   chœur

3. The graphemes **gu** and **qu** can be pronounced three different ways: **[g], [gw], [gɥ]** and **[k], [kw], [kɥ]**, respectively. The majority of words are pronounced with simply **[g]** and **[k]**, but the spelling will not tell you which sound to pronounce, so you'll just have to learn them individually.

[g]	[gw]	[gɥ]	[k]	[kw]	[kɥ]
anguille	jaguar	aiguille	question	adéquat	quiescent
fatigue	iguane	ambiguïté	qualité	aquarium	équilatéral
guérilla	lingual	linguiste	équivalent	square	ubiquité
distinguer	Guadeloupe		quartier	équateur	équidistant

4. Even though most final consonants are not pronounced in French (see below), there are a few exceptions, especially with words ending in -s. In words ending in a consonant + s or -es, the s is silent. However, if a word ends in -as, -ès, -is, -os,

or -us, then the s is sometimes pronounced.

s = silent	*s = pronounced*
cadenas	atlas
débarras	pancréas
accès	aloès
exprès	palmarès
logis	oasis
clos	vis
dessous	albatros
confus	sinus
dehors	ours

Silent Letters

- The final consonant of many words is silent. Sometimes a final c, f, l or r are pronounced though.

  Final c, f, l, r silent

blanc	cléf	outil	parler
franc	cerf	sourcil	chercher
tabac	nerf	gentil	habiter
estomac		persil	fermer

  Final c, f, l, r pronounced

bouc	œuf	fil	car
lac	sauf	avril	mer
avec	veuf	civil	pour
donc	actif	col	hiver

Six Easy Rules for Vowels

A is always ah as in fAther
E ia always A as in Ate
I is always E as in mEat
O is always O as in Over (go figure)
U is always U as in nOOdles.

So there you have it. *Father ate meat over noodles.*

Now for the difficult part. French uses six diacritic marks

The usual diacritic marks are the acute (´ , *accent aigu*), the grave (` , *accent grave*), the circumflex (^ , *circonflexe*), the diaeresis (¨ , *tréma*), and the cedilla (¸ , *cédille*). The Tilde *(cañon)* is also seen. Diacritics have no impact on the primary alphabetical order.

- Acute accent (*é*): Over *e*, indicates uniquely the sound /e/ as in get. An *é* in modern French is often used where a combination of *e* and a consonant, usually *s*, would have been used formerly: *écouter < escouter*.
- Grave accent (*à, è, ù*): Over *a* or *u*, used primarily to distinguish homophones: *à* ("to") vs. *a* ("has"),

ou ("or") vs. *où* ("where"; *ù* exists only in this word). Over an *e*, indicates the sound /ɛ/.

- Circumflex (*â, ê, î, ô, û*): Over *a*, *e* or *o*, indicates the sound /ɑ/, /ɛ/ or /o/, respectively (the distinction *a* /a/ vs. *â* /ɑ/ tends to disappear in Parisian French). Most often indicates the historical deletion of an adjacent letter (usually an *s* or a vowel): *château* < *castel*, *fête* < *feste*, *sûr* < *seur*, *dîner* < *disner*. (In medieval manuscripts many letters were often written as diacritical marks: the circumflex for "s" and the tilde for "n" are examples.) It has also come to be used to distinguish homophones: *du* ("of the") vs. *dû* (past participle of *devoir* "to have to do something (pertaining to an act)"); however *dû* is in fact written thus because of a dropped *e*: *deu*). Since the 1990 orthographic changes, the circumflex on most *i* and *u* may be dropped as there is no change in pronunciation, and it does not serve to distinguish homophones.

- Diaeresis or *tréma* (*ë, ï, ü, ÿ*): Over *e, i, u* or *y*, Indicates that a vowel is to be pronounced separately from the preceding one: *naïve, Noël*. A diaeresis on *y* only occurs in some proper names and in modern editions of old French texts. Some proper names in which *ÿ* appears include *Aÿ* (commune in *canton de la Marne* formerly *Aÿ-Champagne*), *Rue des Cloÿs* (alley in the 18th arrondissement of Paris), *Croÿ* (family name and hotel on the Boulevard Raspail, Paris), *Château du Feÿ* (near Joigny), *Ghÿs* (name of Flemish origin spelt *Ghijs* where *ij* in handwriting looked like *ÿ* to French clerks), *L'Haÿ-les-Roses* (commune between

Paris and Orly airport), Pierre Louÿs (author), Moÿ (place in *commune de l'Aisne* and family name), and *Le Blanc de Nicolaÿ* (an insurance company in eastern France). The diaeresis on *u* appears in the Biblical proper names *Archélaüs, Capharnaüm, Emmaüs, Ésaü* and *Saül,* as well as French names such as Haüy. Nevertheless, since the 1990 orthographic changes, the diaeresis in words containing *guë* (such as *aiguë* or *ciguë*) may be moved onto the *u: aigüe, cigüe,* and by analogy may be used in verbs such as *j'argüe.* In addition, words coming from German retain their Umlaut (*ä, ö* and *ü*) if applicable but use French pronunciation, such as *Kärcher* (trade mark of a pressure washer).

- Cedilla (*ç*): Under *c,* this is pronounced /s/ rather than /k/. Thus *je lance* "I throw" (with *c* = [s] before *e*), *je lançais* "I was throwing" (*c* would be pronounced [k] before *a* without the cedilla). The c cedilla (ç) softens the hard /k/ sound to /s/ before the vowels **a, o** or **u**, for example **ç**a /sa/. *Ç* is never used before the vowels **e, i** or **y** since these three vowels always produce a soft /s/ sound (**ce, ci, cycle**).

The tilde diacritical mark (˜) above n is occasionally used in French for words and names of Spanish origin that have been incorporated into the language (e.g. *cañon, El Niño*). Like the other diacritics, the tilde has no impact on the primary alphabetical order.

Diacritics are often omitted on capital letters, mainly for technical reasons. It is widely believed that they are not required; however both the Académie française and the

Office québécois de la langue française reject this usage and confirm that "in French, the accent has full orthographic value",[1]—except for acronyms but not for abbreviations (e.g. *CEE, ALENA,* but *É.-U.*).

---

[1]   http://en.wikipedia.org/wiki/French_alphabet#cite_note-1

Vowels and Diphthongs (non-nasalized)

A fundamental property of French vowels is that their sounds often depend very much on what consonants happen to be nearby. The proximity of *m* or *n* creates a very special situation which is discussed in the next section; we describe the other cases first.

a	**ah**
ai, ay	**ay**, like English
ail	**iy**, like the word "eye"
ais, ait (final)	**eh**
au	**o**, approximately
e (usually)	**uh**, somewhere between the **e** in English "per" and the **oo** in English "book"; almost a schwa
e (final)	**silent**, except when it follows *r* or *l* or *n* (which in turn must follow something other than *r* or *l* or *n*): then *e* is pronounced as **uh** but is very short, and the previous syllable is stressed, e.g. *quatre* = **kah-truh**
é	**ay**
è, ê	**eh**
eau	**o**, approximately

er, et, ez, eil (final)	**ay** (exception: *La Mer* = **lah mehr**)
eu	**ö**, similar to German: like **ay** but with lips rounded to produce an **oh**-like sound, e.g. *Jeux* = **zhö**
i, ie	**ee**
il, ille (final)	**ee**
o	**oh** (a bit shorter)
oeu	**ö**, basically the same as *eu*
oi	**wah**, e.g. *L'Oiseau Lyre* = **lwah-zoh <u>leer</u>**
ou	**oo** as in "root"
oui	**wee**
u	**ü**, similar to German: like **ee** but with lips rounded to produce an **oo**-like sound, e.g. *Henri Dutilleux* = **a^{n}-ree dü-tee-<u>yö</u>**
ue (final)	**silent**, as in English "vague"
ui	**wee**
y	**ee**

Nasalized Vowels

Certain vowels change slightly when followed by any undoubled *n* or *m* that is not followed by a vowel; in these cases also the *m* or *n* is not fully articulated (unless another consonant follows). The table below lists the most important examples for radio purposes.

an, am	o^n, o^m, e.g. *Nadia Boulanger* = **nah-dee-a boo-lo^n-<u>zhay</u>** , *Estampes* = **es-<u>tomp</u>**
aen	e^n, e.g. *Olivier Messiaen* = **oh-lee-vee-yay mess-see-<u>e</u>^{n}** _____
en, em	**ah^n, ah^m**, e.g. *Charpentier* = **shar-pahn-<u>tyay</u>** , *Vincent D'Indy* = **va^n-sah^n dan-<u>dee</u>** _____
ean	**ah^n**, e.g. *Jean-Yves Thibaudet* = **zhahn-eev tee-boh-<u>day</u>** _____
in, im	**a^n, a^m**, e.g. *François Couperin* = **fro^n-swah koo-per-<u>a</u>^{n}** ◁≡ _____
un, um	**uh^n, uh^m**, e.g. *D'un Soir Triste* = **du^n swahr treest** ◁≡ _____

Vowels in French are pure vowels, i.e. they are not diphthongs as in American English. Americans pronounce a and e with an extra *yuh* sound at the end, and o and u with an extra *wuh* sound at the end. You must not do this in French! The distinction between long and short vowels exists in French, but a few American short vowels do not exist ([ɪ] as in *did* and [ʊ] as in *put*) so make sure to never pronounce these vowels when speaking French. Also notice that the [æ] sound in *cat* does not exist in French.

Vowels in Contrast

Long Vowels	Short Vowels	Similar English
[a]	**[ə]**	*not - nut*
[i]	----	*sheep*
[e]	**[ɛ]**	*wait - wet*
[o]	**[ɔ]**	*coat - caught*
[u]	----	*moon*

On the other hand, French has three front rounded vowels that do not exist in English, which may take a while to get used to since English only has back rounded vowels. However, they are the rounded counterpart of vowels that do exist in English, so you simply need to round your lips when pronouncing these vowels.

Vowels in Contrast

Unrounded	Rounded
[i]	**[y]**
[e]	**[ø]**
[ɛ]	**[œ]**

Many English speakers tend to say **[u]** instead of **[y]** and **[ə]** instead of **[ø]** or **[œ]**.

Words in Contrast

[u] - [y] sous su
[ə] - [ø] ce   ceux

[ø]   - jeûn
[œ]   e   **jeune**

- Similar to English, the final -e in most words is not pronounced. For feminine adjectives and nouns, this generally means that the final consonant of the masculine form will now be pronounced.

Masculine	Feminine
vert	ver**te**
grand	gran**d**e
canadien	canadie**nn**e
boulanger	boulang**è**re
chat	cha**tt**e

- As mentioned above, a few silent letters were placed in French orthography for the prestige of being more similar to Latin. Other letters are now silent for other historical reasons (i.e. perhaps the pronunciation changed, but the spelling did not.) The following words all have silent letters:

sep**t**	ran**g**	fi**ls**	tro**p**
rom**pt**	san**g**	pou**ls**	cam**p**
aspe**ct**	œ**il**	saou**l**	chocola**t**

instin**ct**	fauteui**l**	cu**l**	cré**dit**
pie**d**	ai**l**	Renau**lt**	ri**z**
ni**d**	dra**p**	siro**p**	ne**z**

- A few plural nouns change their pronunciations to include silent letters, whereas these consonants are pronounced in the singular form:

un œuf	des œu**fs**
un bœuf	des bœu**fs**
un os	des o**s**

e caduc

La loi des trois consonnes states that [ə] may be omitted in pronunciation as long as it would not cause three consonants to be together. Of course there are exceptions to this rule, and some dialects of French do not delete it anyway (such as in the south of France.) However, this is extremely common in everyday French and English speakers need to be able to comprehend words with dropped syllables.

Phrase-final e is always dropped, except in -le in the imperative. It is also dropped at the end of nouns, articles and verbs. One exception to the three consonant rule is in the case of consonant clusters, such as br, fr, gr, pr, tr, etc. If the e precedes these clusters, and the e itself is preceded by a consonant, then it can be dropped: un refrain = un r'frain

Disappearing e

Careful Speech	*Normal Speech*
samedi / lentement / sauvetage	*/ sam'di / lent'ment / sauv'tage*
sous le bureau / chez le docteur	*sous l'bureau / chez l'docteur*
il y a de / pas de / plus de	*il y a d' / pas d' / plus d'*
je ne / de ne / tu ne	*je n' / de n' / tu n'*
je te / ce que / ce qui	*j'te / c'que / c'qui*

Notice that dropping e in *je* also results in [ʒ] to become [ʃ] whenever it is found before voiceless consonants, such as [p], [t], [k], etc.

Liaison

A loss of word boundaries in French makes it difficult to comprehend the spoken language for beginning learners. All of the words seem to be linked together without any clear divisions because the syllable boundaries do not correspond to the word boundaries. In many cases, the last consonant from one syllable (which is usually silent) will become the first consonant of the next syllable (therefore, it is no longer silent). This linking between syllables is called liaison, and it may or may not be required and the pronunciation of the consonant may or may not change. Liaison leads to many homonymous phrases, which can hinder comprehension. You must pay attention to the liaisons in verb conjugations as well or you may mistake one verb for another.

The consonants involved in liaison generally include d, s, and x. However, their pronunciation is changed so that they become [t], [z] and [z], respectively. The letter n that is written after nasal vowels becomes the nasal consonant [n]. Peculiarly, the f of neuf is pronounced [v] only before *ans* and *heures* and in all other cases, it remains [f]. And remember that h aspiré prevents liaison from happening, i.e. there is no [z] sound between *des* and *haricots*.

Examples of Liaison

elle**s a**rrivent	mo**n a**mour
il**s o**nt	le**s o**urs
vieu**x a**rbres	dan**s u**n sac
di**x h**eures	trè**s a**imable
atten**d-il** ?	plu**s o**uvert
gran**d a**mi	il es**t a**llé

There are a few instances when you should always use liaison (*liaison obligatoire*):

1. after determiners: **un, les, des, ces, mon, ton, quels,** etc.
2. before or after pronouns: **nous, vous, ils, elles, les,** etc.
3. after preceding adjectives: **bon, mauvais, petit, grand, gros,** etc.

4. after monosyllabic prepositions: **chez, dans, sous, en,** etc.
5. after some monosyllabic adverbs: **très, plus, bien,** etc. (optional after pas, trop, fort)
6. after **est** (optional after all other forms of être)

Stress

French is a syllable-timed language, so equal emphasis is given to each syllable. This is quite unlike English, which is a stress-timed language, and which gives emphasis to one syllable in each word - the stressed syllable - and reduces the vowels in the rest of the syllables (usually to [ə] or [ɪ].) All vowels in French must be pronounced fully, and each syllable must be pronounced with equal stress, though the final syllable of each word is generally considered the "stressed syllable."

Listen to these words in English and French and see if you can hear the difference in stress. Stressed syllables in English are marked in bold.

- phot**o**graphy - photographie
- aut**ho**rity - autorité
- natio**na**lity - nationalité
- **pa**ssion - passion
- edu**ca**tion - éducation
- **re**giment - régiment
- **mon**ument - monument
- melodra**ma**tic - mélodramatique

Intonation

Intonation in French is slightly different from English. In general, the intonation rises only for a yes/no question, and the rest of the time, the intonation falls. French intonation starts at a higher pitch and falls continuously throughout the sentence, whereas in English, the stressed syllable has a higher pitch that what precedes and follows it.

Listen to these sentences in English and French and see if you can hear the difference in intonation. Bold marks the higher pitch. Notice that even if the intonation pattern seems similar, the syllables with higher pitches are often in different locations. The numbers below refer to the pitch: 1) low, 2) medium, 3) high, 4) extra high.

English Intonation vs. French Intonation

Sentence Type	English	Intonation	French	Intonation
Yes/No Question	Are you **leaving**?	2 - 3	Est-ce que vous par**tez** ?	2 - 3
Information Question	Where are you **go**ing?	2 - 3 - 1	**Où** est-ce que vous allez ?	4 - 2 - 1
Imperative	**Do** it. / Don't **do** it.	/ (2) - 3 - 1	**Fais**-le. / **Ne** le fais pas.	4 - 2 - 1
Exclamation	What a sur**pri**se!	2 - 3 - 1	**Quelle** surprise !	4 - 2 - 1
Declarative	I bought a	2 - 3 -	**J'ai** acheté	3 - 2 -

dre_ss._   _1_   _une robe._   _1_

Informal Reductions

In everyday speech, there are other reductions in addition to _e caduc._ Many of these reductions are made for ease of pronunciation and are considered informal. The most common ones are reducing tu to t' before a vowel and omitting the final syllable of words ending in -re. Listen to these reductions in careful speech and everyday speech:

Informal Reductions in Spoken French

Careful Speech	_Everyday Speech_
_tu es_	_t'es_
_tu as_	_t'as_
tu étais	_t'étais_
tu avais	_t'avais_
mettre	_mett'_
notre	_not'_
autre	_aut'_
_il_	_y_
_il y a_	_y a_
ils + vowel	_y'z_
elle	_è_
elles + vowel	_è'z_
parce que	_pasq'_

quelque   *quèq'*
puis   *pis*

Sources: http://ielanguages.com/frenchphonetics.html
http://www.pronunciationguide.info/French.html

Introductions – Présentations

Do you speak French?	Parlez-vous français ?
Good day, good evening.	Bonjour, bonsoir (after 7pm).
What is your name?	Comment vous appelez-vous ?
	Comment t'appelles-tu ?
	Quel est votre nom ?
I am nurse/ doctor Smith.	Je suis l'infirmier/ l'infirmière/ le docteur Smith.
I am an anesthetist, a surgeon, a gynecologist, a general practitioner.	Je suis anesthésiste, chirurgien/chirurgienne, gynécologue, généraliste.
I will be performing your anesthesia/surgery.	Je vais faire votre anesthésie/ chirurgie.
My name is Janet.	Je m'appelle Janet.
Yes, I understand.	Oui , je comprends.
I don't understand very	Je ne comprends pas très

well.	bien.
I understand a little.	Je comprends un peu.
I understand almost everything.	Je comprends presque tout.
Do you understand me?	Est-ce que vous me comprenez ?
How do you say "book" in French?	Comment dit-on "book" en français ?
Please speak more slowly.	Parlez plus lentement s'il vous plait.
I'm sorry, I do not understand.	Désolé, je ne comprends pas.
Please repeat slowly.	S'il vous plait, répétez lentement.

General questions - Questions generals

How are you feeling today?	Comment vous sentez-vous, aujourd'hui ?
I have some questions for you.	J'ai quelques questions pour vous.
If possible, answer in a simple way.	Si possible répondez simplement.
How old are you?	Quel âge avez-vous ?
How much do you weigh?	Combien pesez-vous ?
How tall are you?	Combien mesurez-vous ?
Do you have any allergies?	Etes-vous allergique à quelque chose ?
Are you allergic to any medications?	Etes-vous allergique à un médicament en particulier ?
Are you allergic to rubber gloves? (latex)	Etes-vous allergique aux gants en caoutchouc ?

Do you take any medications?	Est-ce que vous prenez des médicaments ?
What medicines?	Quels sont les noms des médicaments ?
What are the medications for?	Les médicaments sont pour quoi ?
Do you smoke? How many cigarettes each day?	Fumez-vous ? Combien de cigarettes par jour ?
Do you drink alcohol? How much?	Est-ce que vous buvez de l'alcool ? Combien?
Do you take or have you ever taken drugs?	Est-ce que vous prenez ou avez pris des drogues ?
Is there any chance you could be pregnant?	Est-ce qu'il y a un risque que vous soyez enceinte ?

Ache and illnesses – Douleurs et maladies

Presently do you have a cold?	Maintenant, avez-vous un rhume ?
Do you have a fever?	Est-ce que vous avez de la fièvre ?
Do you cough?	Est-ce que vous toussez ?
Do you have a stuffy nose?	Est-ce que vous avez le nez bouché ?
Are you hurting somewhere?	Avez-vous mal quelque part ?
Does your... hurt? - use with the words below.	Avez-vous mal à ….
	… mal à la tête (headache) , aux oreilles (ears) , au nez (nose), aux sinus (sinus), aux dents (teeth), à la bouche (mouth), à la gorge (throat), au cou (neck), au dos (back), aux reins (lower

	back, kidney region), à la poitrine (chest and breasts), à l'estomac (stomach), au foie (liver), au sexe (pelvis), à l'anus (anus), aux bras (arms), aux mains (hands), aux doigts (fingers), aux articulations (joints), aux jambes (legs), aux genoux (knees), aux chevilles (ankles), aux pieds (feet), aux orteils (toes).
Can you point at where it hurts?	Pouvez-vous me montrer avec votre doigt où vous avez mal ?
Do you have skin problems?	Est-ce que vous avez des problèmes de peau ?
Do you have pimples? Rashes? Does anything itch?	Est-ce que vous avez des boutons ? Des éruptions cutanées ? Est-ce que ça vous gratte quelque part ?
Do you have parasites, worms, lice, fleas?	st-ce que vous avez des parasites, des vers, des poux, des puces ?
Do you eat well?	Est-ce que vous mangez bien ?

Are you depressed? Do you take anti-depressive medicines?	Est-ce que vous êtes déprimé ? Est-ce que vous prenez des anti-dépressifs ?
Do you have hearing problems?	Avez-vous des problèmes d'audition ?
Do you have eye problems?	15. Avez-vous des problèmes de vision ?
Do you faint?	16. Est-ce que vous vous évanouissez ?
Have you had hepatitis?	17. Avez-vous eu une hépatite ?
Have you had malaria? How many times? When?	18. Avez-vous eu le paludisme ? Combien de fois ? Quand ?
Are you diabetic? Do you take medications for it?	19. Avez-vous du diabète ? Prenez-vous des médicaments pour ça ?
Do you have problems with your thyroid?	20. Avez-vous des problèmes avec votre tyroïde ?

Have you ever had seizures?	21. Avez-vous eu des attaques d'épilepsie ?
Have you ever been diagnosed with cancer? If so which type?	22. Avez-vous eu un cancer ? Si oui, quel type ?
When you get a cut do you bleed normally or more than other people?	23. Quand vous vous coupez, est-ce que vous saignez normalement ou plus que les autres ?
Have you had a blood transfusion? When?	24. Est-ce que vous avez eu des transfusions sanguines ? Quand ?
Do you have AIDS?	25. Avez-vous le SIDA ?
Have you been tested for AIDS?	26. Avez-vous été testé pour le SIDA ?

Cardiovascular system – Système cardiovasculaire

Do you have any problems with your blood pressure?	Avez-vous un problème de tension artérielle ?
Do you have problems with your heart?	Avez-vous des problèmes cardiaques ?
What kind of problem?	Quelle sorte de problèmes ?
Have you had a heart attack? Stroke? When?	Est-ce que vous avez eu des attaques cardiaques ? des attaques cérébrales ? Quand ?
Do you take any medecine for these problems?	Prenez-vous des médicaments pour ces problèmes ?

Pulmonary system – Système pulmonaire

Do you have asthma?	Avez-vous de l'asthme ?
Do you have respiratory problems?	Avez-vous des problèmes pulmonaires ou respiratoires ?
Do you take any medecine for these problems?	Prenez-vous des médicaments pour ces problèmes ?
Have you had tubeculosis? When? Did you take medication?	Avez-vous eu la tuberculose ? Quand ? Avez-vous pris des medicaments ?

System gastointestinal – Système gastro-intestinal

Does it hurt when you go to the bathroom?	Est-ce que vous avez mal lorsque vous allez aux toilettes ?
Is there blood in your pee or your stools?	Est-ce qu'il y a du sang dans vos urines ou dans vos selles ?
Do you have diarrhea?	Avez-vous la diarrhée ?
Are you constipated?	Êtes-vous constipé ?
When you lie down does acid or food come up into your mouth?	Quand vous êtes allongé, est-ce que vous avez de l'acide ou de la nourriture qui remonte dans votre gorge ?
Are you nauseous?	Est-ce que vous avez la nausée ?
Are you vomiting?	Est-ce que vous vomissez ?
Do you have parasites, worms?	Est-ce que vous avez des parasites, des vers ?

System urogenital - Système uro-génital

Is there blood in your pee or your stools?	Est-ce qu'il y a du sang dans vos urines ou dans vos selles ?
Do you have a sexually transmissible disease?	Est-ce que vous avez une maladie sexuellement transmissible ?
Have you had a blood transfusion? When?	Est-ce que vous avez eu des transfusions sanguines ? Quand ?
Are you HIV positive?	Avez-vous le SIDA ?
Have you been tested for HIV?	Avez-vous été testé pour le SIDA ?

For women - Pour les femme

Do you have regular periods?	Est-ce que vos règles sont régulières ?
Are you taking a birth control pill?	Est-ce que vous prenez la pilule ?
Have you ever been pregnant?	Avez-vous déjà été enceinte ?
How many pregnancies have you had?	Combien de grossesses avez-vous eu ?
How many children do you have?	Combien d'enfants avez-vous ?
When was the birth?	Quand avez-vous accouché ?
Did you have anesthesia for the delivery?	Est-ce que vous avez eu une anesthésie pour votre accouchement ?
What sort of anesthesia did you have?	Quelle sorte d'anesthésie avez-vous eue ?

Physical exam - Examen physique

Now, I'm going to take your temperature.	Maintenant, je vais prendre votre température.
I'm going to take your blood pressure.	Je vais prendre votre pression sanguine/artérielle.
I'm going to measure you, to weigh you.	Je vais vous mesurer/vous peser.
Respirez profondément.	Il faut que j'écoute vos poumons.
I'm going to look at your ears and your eyes.	Je vais regarder vos oreilles et vos yeux.
I'm going to look at your mouth, your teeth, your tongue. Open your mouth please. Stick your tongue out.	Je vais regarder votre bouche, vos dents, votre langue. Ouvrez la bouche s'il vous plaît. Tirez la langue s'il vous plaît.
If you allow me, I have to do a pelvic exam.	Si vous le permettez, je dois regarder votre sexe.
I have to give you a shot.	Il faut que je vous fasse une piqûre.

We have to run more tests.	Il faut faire plus de tests.
	Une radio (an X-ray). Une analyse de sang (a blood analysis). Une analyse de sang (a blood analysis). Une analyse d'urine/ de selles (urine/stool analysis). Un electrocardiogramme (ECG).
Don't move.	Ne bougez pas.
Slide toward me.	Glissez vers moi.
Sit down.	Asseyez-vous.
Lie down on your right/left/ on your back (supine)/on your stomach (prone).	Couchez-vous sur le côté droit/gauche/ sur le dos/ sur le ventre.
Squeeze my hand.	Pressez ma main.
Open/close your mouth.	Ouvrez/Fermez la bouche.
Swallow.	Déglutissez (avalez).
Cough.	Toussez.

I am an anesthetist (surgeon/gynecologist/general practitioner).	Je suis anesthésiste. (chirurgien/chirurgienne/ gynécologue/généraliste).
I will be performing your anesthesia.	Je vais faire votre anesthésie.
What operation are you having today ?	Quelle opération avez-vous aujourd'hui ?
With your finger point to where they will operate on you.	Montrez- moi avec votre doigt où ils vont vous opérer.
Are you allergic to any medications ?	Etes-vous allergique à un médicament en particulier ?
Are you allergic to rubber gloves ?	Etes-vous allergique aux gants en caoutchouc ?
What operations have you had ?	Quelles opérations avez-vous eues ?
What sort of anesthesia have you had ?	Quelles sortes d'anesthésies avez-vous eues ?

General anesthesia ?	Anesthésie générale ?
Spinal anesthesia ?	Anesthésie rachidienne ? (de la colonne vertébrale ?
Local anesthesia ?	Anesthésie locale ?
How much do you weigh ? How tall are you ?	Combien pesez-vous ? Combien mesurez-vous ?
Have you or a member of your family had any problems with anesthesia ?	Est-ce que vous, ou un membre de votre famille, a eu des problèmes avec l'anesthésie ?
When did you last have anything to eat ?	Quand avez-vous mangé pour la dernière fois ?
You must arrive for surgery fasting.	Il faut que vous arriviez pour votre chirurgie à jeun.
How many hours has it been since you had anything to eat or drink ? one, two, three, four, five, six, seven, eight or more ?	Il y a combien d'heures depuis que vous avez mangé ou bu quelque chose ? Une, deux, trois, quatre, cinq, six, sept, huit, ou plus ?
Do this. Tilt your head back like this.	Faites ça. Penchez la tête un peu derrière comme ça.

Turn your head to the right and left.	Tournez votre tête de droite à gauche.
Open your mouth. Close your mouth.	Ouvrez la bouche. Fermez la bouche.
Stick out your tongue	Tirez la langue.
Show me your teeth.	Montrez-moi vos dents.
Do you have teeth that move, are broken, or false teeth that come out ?	Avez-vous des dents qui bougent, cassées, ou de fausses dents qui pourraient tomber ?
If yes, you need to take them out before surgery.	Si oui, vous devez les retirer avant la chirurgie.
Have you taken any medications today ?	Avez-vous pris des médicaments aujourd'hui ?
I have to listen to your lungs. Breathe deeply. In and out, hold your breath. Breathe normally.	Il faut que j'écoute vos poumons. Respirez profondément. Inspirez, expirez, retenez votre respiration. Respirez normalement.

Sometimes there are complications of anesthesia, but they are very rare, and we will take very good care of you.	Quelques fois, il y a des complications à cause de l'anesthésie, mais c'est très rare, et nous nous occuperons bien de vous.
Informed consent	**Permission pour la procédure**
This document explains the surgery and anesthesia and their risks.	Ce document contient une explication de la chirurgie et de l'anesthésie, et des risques.
Please read the document.	S'il vous plait, lisez ce document.
Do you need someone to read the document to you ?	Avez-vous besoin que quelqu'un vous lise le document ?
Do you understand it ?	Est-ce que vous le comprenez ?
Do you agree to go ahead with the surgery.	Est-ce que vous êtes d'accord pour faire l'opération ?
Please put your signature and the	S'il vous plait, signez et

date, here.	mettez la date d'aujourd'hui ici.

Surgery | ## Opération

I have to start an intravenous infusion to give you fluid and medicine.	Il faut que je commence une perfusion pour vous donner des fluides et des médicaments.
I will be giving you some medicines through the intravenous and you will fall asleep.	Je vais vous donner des médicaments à travers votre perfusion, et vous allez vous endormir.
When the operation is finishing you will awaken.	Quand l'opération sera finie, vous vous réveillerez.
	Quand vous vous réveillerez, il est possible que vous ayez un peu mal à la gorge. C'est normal, et ça va passer.
	Anesthésie rachidienne. Après une petite piqûre dans le bas du dos, vous serez insensible et donc vous ne

	sentirez pas l'opération.
Do you feel anything in your legs.	Sentez-vous quelque chose dans vos jambes ?
Do your legs feel warm ?	Est-ce que vos jambes sont chaudes ?
Do your legs feel normal ?	Est-ce que vos jambes sont normales ?
Do your legs feel numb ?	Est-ce que vos jambes sont engourdies ?
Is there a metallic taste in your mouth ?	Est-ce que vous avez un goût métallique dans la bouche ?
Do you feel this ?	Est-ce que vous sentez ça ?
Ou la même chose ?	Est-ce que c'est plus fort ici, ou là ?
If you prefer you can sleep during the operation.	Si vous préférez, vous pouvez dormir pendant l'opération.
We will take you into the operating room now.	Nous allons vous emmener dans la salle d'opération maintenant.

Go there	Mettez-vous là.
Slide a little toward me.	Glissez un peu vers moi.
Move down a bit.	Descendez un peu.
Move up a little on the table.	Remontez un peu sur la table.
Lie down.	Couchez-vous.
Lie down on your right/left side.	Couchez-vous sur le côté droit/gauche.
Lie down on your back/stomach.	Couchez-vous sur le dos/ sur le ventre.
Give me your arm.	Donnez-moi votre bras.
Don't move.	Ne bougez pas.
Relax.	Détendez-vous.
Raise your head.	Levez la tête.
Lower your head.	Baissez la tête.

English	French
You will feel a little pressure.	Vous allez sentir un peu de pression.
I am taking your blood pressure.	Je prends votre pression sanguine (artérielle).
Open your eyes.	Ouvrez les yeux.
Close your eyes.	Fermez les yeux.
Ça ne va pas vous déranger.	Je vais vous donner un peu d'oxygène à travers ce masque.
Breathe deeply.	Respirez profondément.
Nous allons bien nous occuper de vous.	Ne vous inquiétez pas.
Now you will feel sleepy.	Maintenant, vous allez avoir sommeil.
You will fall asleep.	Vous allez vous endormir maintenant.
Post anesthesia	**Après l'opération**
The operation is finished.	L'opération est finie.

Please cough.	Toussez s'il vous plait.
Squeeze my hand.	Pressez ma main – plus fort.
Lift your legs.	Levez les jambes.
Sit down.	Asseyez-vous.
Bend your knees.	Pliez les genoux.
This will feel cold.	Ça va être froid.
You will feel a little pinch.	Vous allez sentir un petit pincement.
Do you feel anything in your legs ?	Sentez-vous quelque chose dans vos jambes ?
Do you feel dizzy ?	Est-ce que vous avez la tête qui tourne ?
Can you move your feet ?	Pouvez-vous bouger vos pieds ?
Can you move your toes ?	Pouvez-vous remuer les doigts de pied ?

We are going to raise your legs.	Nous allons lever vos jambes.
Do you have discomfort ?	Avez-vous mal ?
Now do you have more or less discomfort ?	Et maintenant vous avez moins ou plus mal ?
Are you nauseated ?	Avez-vous mal au coeur ? (la nausée)
Do you have chest pain ?	Est-ce que vous avez mal à la poitrine ?
We will give you medicine so that you feel less sick.	Nous allons vous donner des médicaments pour que vous ayez moins mal.
Spinal headache	**Migraine post opératoire**
Do you have a headache ?	Avez-vous mal à la tête ?
Is it worse when you sit up or lie down ?	Est-ce que vous avez plus mal quand vous êtes assis ou allongé ?

You need to drink a lot of water to make the headache better.	Vous devez boire beaucoup d'eau pour guérir votre mal de tête.

English - Français

~ A ~

Abacterial - (Abactérien)
Abdomen - (Abdomen)
Abdominal - (Abdominal)
Abdominal muscle contraction - (Contraction muscles abdominaux)
Abdominocentesis - (Abdominocentèse)
Abdominogenital - (Abdominogénital)
Abduction - (Abduction)
Aberrant - (Aberrant)
Aberration - (Aberration)
Ablaction - (Ablactation)
Ablation - (Ablation)
Able, to be - (Pouvoir)
Abnormal - (Anormal)
Abnormal - (Anormal)
Abnormality - (Anormalité)
abomasum - (caillette)
Abort; miscarry, to - (Avorter)
Aborted - (Avorté(e))
Abortifacient - (Abortif (tive))
abortion - (l'avortement)
Abortion rate - (Taux d'avortement)
Abortion; miscarriage - (Avortement)
Above - (En haut)

Abrasion - (Abrasion)
Abrupt - (Abrupt (e))
abscess - (abcès)
Absence - (Absence)
Absorption - (Absorption)
Abstemious - (Abstème)
Abstinence - (Abstinence)
Abundant - (Abondant)
Abuse - (Abus)
Academic - (Académique)
acaricide - (acaricide)
Access - (Accès)
Accident - (Accident)
accident - (choc)
Accident, to have an - (Avoir un accident)
Accident; crash - (Accidenter)
Accidents at home - (Accident domestiques)
Accommodate, to; adjust, to - (Accommoder)
Accommodation - (Accommodation)
Accomplishment - (Accomplissement)
Accumulation - (Accumulation)
Accustomed - (Habitué(e))
Acetabulum - (Acétabule)
Acetone - (Acétone)
Acetonuria - (Acétonurie)
Acetylcholine - (Acetylcholine)
Acid - (Acide)

Acidemia - (Acidose)
Acidity - (Acidité)
Acidosis - (Acidose)
Acinus - (Acinus)
Acne - (Acné)
Acrocyanosis - (Acrocyanose)
Acromegaly - (Acromégalie)
Acromion - (Acromion)
Act, to - (Agir)
ACTH - (ACTH)
Activator - (Activeur)
Active - (Actif(ve))
Activity - (Activité)
Actuation - (Conduite, façon d'agir)
Acuity - (Acuité)
Acupuncture - (Acupuncture)
Acute - (Grave)
acute disease - (maladie aiguë)
Acute hepatitis - (Hépatite aiguë)
Acyclovir - (Activir)
Acyclovir - (zovirax)
Adaptation - (Adaptation)
Addiction - (Dépendance)
Adduction - (Adduction)
Adductor - (Adducteur)
Adenitis - (Adénite)
Adenocarcinoma - (Adénocarcinome)
Adenoid - (Adénoïde)
Adenoid - (Adénoïdien)
Adenoidectomy - (Adénoïdectomie)

Adenoiditis - (Adénoïdite)
Adenoma - (Adénome)
Adenopathy - (Adénopathie)
Adequate - (Adéquat(e))
Adhesion - (Adhérence)
adipose - (Adipose)
Adjacent organ - (Organe ajouté (e, es))
Adjust, to - (Ajuster)
Administration - (Administration)
Admission - (Admission)
Admission of patients - (Admission de patients)
Adnexa - (Organe ajouté (e, es))
Adolescence - (Adolescence)
Adolescent - (Adolescent)
Adrenal - (Adrénergique)
Adrenaline - (Adrénaline)
Adrenocorticotropin - (Adrénocorticotropine)
Adult - (Adulte)
Adulterated - (Falsifié(e))
Adulteration - (Falsification)
Advance - (Avance, progrès)
Adverse - (Adverse, contraire)
Adverse drug reaction, ADR - (Réaction adverse à un médicament, RAM)
Adverse effect - (Effet adverse)
Adverse effects - (Effets nocifs)
Advice; counsel - (Conseil)

Advisable - (Conseillé(e))
Adynamia - (Asthénie, adynamie)
Aerobe - (Aérobie)
Aerogastria - (Aérogastrie)
Aerophagia - (Aérophagie)
Aerosol - (Aérosol)
Afebrile - (Sans fièvre)
Affected by a heart condition - (Affecté au cœur)
Affected by AIDS - (Affectés par le SIDA)
Affection - (Affection)
Afferent - (Afférent)
Affinity - (Affinité)
Affliction - (Affliction)
Afternoon; early evening - (Tard, après midi)
Against - (Contre)
Agalorrhea - (Agalactie)
Age - (Age)
Age, to - (Vieillir)
Agenesis - (Agénésie)
Agent - (Agent)
Agglutination - (Agglutination)
Agglutinogen - (Agglutinogène)
Aggressive - (Agressif (ve))
Agitate, to - (Agiter)
agitation - (Agitation)
Agranulocytosis - (Agranulocytose)
Agree, to - (Accorder)
Agreement - (Accord)
Ahead - (En avant, progresser)

AIDS - (SIDA)
Air - (Air)
Alarm - (Alarme)
Alarming - (Alarmant, inquiétant)
Albino - (Albinos)
Albumin - (Albumine)
Albuminuria - (Albuminurie)
Alcohol - (Alcool)
alcoholemy - (Alcoolémie)
Alcoholic - (Alcoolique)
Alcoholism - (Alcoolisme)
Aldosterone - (Aldostérone)
Alert - (Alerte)
alfalfa - (luzerne)
Algia - (Algie)
Algorhithm - (Algorithme)
Alive - (Vivant (e))
Alkaloid - (Alcaloïde)
Alkalosis - (Alcalose)
All - (Tout)
Allantois - (Allantoïdes)
Allergen - (Allergène)
Allergic - (Allergique)
Allergist - (Allergologiste)
Allergy - (Allergie)
Alleviate - (Soulager)
Alleviate pain - (Soulagement de la douleur)
Alone; only - (Seul (e))
Alopecia - (Alopécie)
Alpha fetoprotein - (Alpha fœto- protéine)
Alter - (Altérer)
Alter - (changer)
Alter - (modifier)

Alter - (troubler)
Alternative - (Alternative)
Alveolar - (Alvéolaire)
Alveolitis - (Alvéolite)
Alveolus - (Alvéole)
Always - (Toujours)
Amalgam - (Amalgame)
Amaurosis - (Amaurose)
Amblyopia - (Amblyopie)
Ambulance - (Ambulance)
Ambulatory - (Ambulatoire, dispensaire)
Ambulatory care - (Soin ambulatoire)
Ameba - (Amibe)
Amebiasis - (Amibiase)
Amenorreha - (Aménorrhée)
Ametropia - (Amétropie)
Amino acids - (Aminoacides)
Amino acids, Essential - (Aminoacides essentiels)
Amnesia - (Amnésie)
Amnesiac - (Amnésique)
Amniocentesis - (Amniocentèse)
Amnios - (Amnios)
Amniotic - (Amniotique)
Amniotic fluid - (Liquide amniotique)
Amoebic dysentery - (Dysenterie amibienne)
Amphetamine - (Amphétamine)
Ampicilin - (Ampicilline)
Amputate - (Amputer)

Amputation - (Amputation)
Amylase - (Amylase)
Anabolic - (Anabolisant)
anaemia - (anémie)
Anaerobic - (Anaérobie)
Anaerobiosis - (Anaérobiose)
anaesthetic - (anesthésique)
Anal - (Anal)
Analgesia - (Analgésie)
Analgesic - (Analgésique)
Analogic - (Analogue)
Analysis - (Analyse)
Analyze - (Analyser)
Anaphylactic - (Anaphylactique)
Anaphylactic shock - (Choc anaphylactique)
Anaphylaxis - (Anaphylaxie)
Anasarca - (Anasarque)
Anastomosis - (Anastomose)
Anatomic - (Anatomique)
Anatomy - (Anatomie)
Androgenous - (Androgène)
Androgenous - (Androgène)
Anemia - (Anémie)
Anemia, Sickle cell - (Anémie falciforme)
Anemic - (Anémique, anémié)
Anencephaly - (Anencéphale)
Anergy - (Anergie)
Anesthesia - (Anesthésie)
Anesthesiologist - (Anesthésiste)
Anesthetic - (Anesthésique)
Anesthetize - (Anesthésier)

Aneurysm - (Anévrisme)
Angina - (Angine)
Angina pectoris - (Angine de poitrine)
Angina, unstable - (Angine instable)
Angioedema - (Angio oedème)
Angiography - (Angiographie)
Angioma - (Angiome)
Angioplasty - (Angioplastie)
Angiospasm - (Vasospasme)
Angitis - (Angéite)
anguish - (Agonie)
Animal - (Animal)
Anisocoria - (Aniscorie)
Ankle - (Cheville)
Ankylosed - (Ankylosé)
Ankylosis - (Ankylose)
Anorexia - (Anorexie)
Anosmia - (Anosmie)
Anovulatory - (Anovulatoire)
Anoxia - (Anoxie)
Antacid - (Antiacide)
Antagonism - (Antagonisme)
Antecubital - (Ante cubital)
Anterior - (Antérieur)
Anterior fontanel - (Fontanelle antérieure)
Anthelmintic - (Antihelminthique)
Anthrax - (Anthrax)
Anti-allergic - (Antiallergique)
Antiarrhythmic - (Anti arythmique)
Anti-asthmatic - (Antiasthmatique)

Antibacterial - (Antimicrobien)
Antibiogram - (Antibiogramme)
Antibiotic - (Antibiotique)
antibiotic - (antibiotique)
Antibody - (Anticorps)
antibody - (anticorps)
Anti-cancer - (Anticancéreux)
Anticoagulant - (Anticoagulant)
Anticonvulsive - (Anti convulsif (ve))
Antidepressant - (Anti dépressif)
Anti-diarrhea - (Anti diarrhéique)
Antidote - (Antidote)
Antiemetic - (Antiémétique)
Anti-flu - (Antigrippal)
Anti-flu medication with paracetamol - (Médicament contra la grippeavec paracétamol)
Antifungal - (Antifongique)
Antigen - (Antigène)
antigen - (antigène)
Antihistamine - (Antihistaminique)
Antihypertensive - (Anti hypertenseur (se))
Anti-inflamatory - (Anti inflammatoire)
Antimigrainous - (Antimigraineux)
Anti-motion sickness - (Contre le mal de mer)

Antineoplastic - (Antinéoplasique)
Antiparasitic - (Antiparasitaire)
Antiplatelet - (Antiagrégant plaquettaire)
Anti-polio - (Antipoliomyélitique)
Antipyretic - (Antipyrétique)
Antiretroviral - (Antirétroviral)
Antisepsis - (Antisepsie)
Antiseptic - (Antiseptique)
antiseptic - (antiseptique)
antiserum - (antisérum)
Antispasmodic - (Antispasmodique)
Antitoxin - (Antitoxine)
Antituberculous - (Antituberculeux)
Antivariolic - (Antivariolique)
antiviral - (activir)
Antiviral - (Antiviral)
Antiviral - (Antivirus)
antiviral - (zovirax)
Anuria - (Anurie)
Anus - (Anus)
anus - (anus)
Anvil; incus - (Enclume)
Anxiety - (Angoisse)
Anxiety - (Anxiété)
Anxious - (Agité(e))
Anxious - (Anxieux)
Aorta - (Aorte)
Aortic - (Aortique)
Aphasia - (Aphasie)
Aphonia; loss of voice -

(Aphonie)
Aphonic - (Aphone)
Aphrodisiac - (Aphrodisiaque)
Aphtha; small ulcer - (Aphte)
Apicectomy - (Apicectomie)
Aplasia - (Aplasie)
Apnea - (Apnée)
Aponeurosis - (Aponévrose)
Apophysis - (Apophyse)
Apoplexy - (Apoplexie)
Apoplexy - (Apoplexie)
Apoplexy, embolic - (Apoplexie embolique)
Apoplexy, hemorrhagic - (Apoplexie hémorragique)
Appearance - (Apparence)
Appearance; features - (Physionomie)
Appendicitis - (Appendicite)
Appendix - (Appendice)
Appetite - (Appétit)
Applicator - (Applicateur)
Apply - (Appliquer)
Appropriate - (Approprié(e))
Approximately - (Approximativement)
Aqueous - (Solution aqueuse)
Aqueous humor - (Humeur aqueuse)
Arbovirus - (Arbovirus)
ARDS - (Syndrome respiratoire)
Areflexia - (Absence de réflexe)
Areola - (Aréole)

Areola (women) / nipple (men); baby bottle/pacifier - (Mamelon)

Arm - (Bras)

Armpit - (Aisselle)

Arrest (as in cardiac or respiratory arrest) - (Arrêt)

Arrest, cardiac - (Arrêt cardiaque)

Arrest, respiratory - (Arrêt respiratoire)

Arrhythmia - (Arythmie)

Arteriosclerosis - (Artériosclérose)

Artery - (Artère)

artery - (artère)

Arthralgia - (Arthralgie)

Arthritic - (Arthritique)

Arthritis - (Arthrite)

arthritis - (arthrite)

Arthroscopy - (Arthroscopie)

Arthrosis - (Arthrose)

Articular capsule - (Capsule articulaire)

Artificial - (Artificiel)

Ascariasis - (Ascaridiase)

Ascariasis - (Ascaridiose)

Ascendance - (Ascendance)

Ascites - (Ascite)

Ascorbic acid - (Acide ascorbique)

Asepsis - (Asepsie)

Aseptic - (Aseptique)

Asexual chromosome - (Chromosome asexuel)

Asphyxia - (Étouffement)

Asphyxiate - (Étouffer)

Aspirate - (Aspirer)

Aspiration - (Aspiration)

Aspirin - (Aspirine)

Assist - (Soigner)

Assist; attend - (Assister)

Assistance - (Assistance)

Assistant - (Aide)

Association - (Association)

Asthenia - (Asthénie)

Asthma - (Asthme)

Asthmatic - (Asthmatique)

Astigmatism - (Astigmatisme)

Astringent - (Astringent)

Asylum; psychiatric hospital - (Asile des aliénés)

Asymmetrical - (Asymétrique)

Asymptomatic - (Asymptomatique)

Ataxia - (Ataxie)

Atelactasis - (Atélectasie)

Atheroma - (Athérome)

Athetosis - (Athétose)

Atomizer - (Atomiseur)

Atresia - (Atrésie)

Atrial fibrillation - (Fibrillation auriculaire)

Atrial flutter - (Tachycardie auriculaire)

Atrioventricular - (Atrioventriculaire)

Atrophy - (Atrophie)

Atropine - (Atropine)

Attack - (Crise)

Attack, Heart, to have a - (Avoir une crise cardiaque)

Attendent; assistant - (Assistant)
Auditory - (Auditif)
Aunt - (Tante)
Aura - (Aura)
Aural - (Relatif à l'aura)
Auricle (of external ear) - (Pavillon de l'oreille)
Auricular - (Auriculaire)
Auscultate - (Ausculter)
Auscultation - (Auscultation)
Auto-immune - (Auto-immune)
Automatism - (Automatisme)
Autonomous - (Autonome)
Autopsy - (Autopsie)
Autopsy - (Nécropsie)
Autosomatic - (Autosome)
Availability - (Disponibilité)
Avitaminosis - (Avitaminose)
Avitaminosis - (Hypovitaminose)
Awake - (Eveillé)
axilla - (aisselle)
Axon - (Axone)
Azoospermia - (Azoospermie)
Azotemia - (Azotémie)

~ B ~

B.I.D.; twice a day - (Deux fois par jour)
Baby - (Bébé)
Baby - (Bebé, Nouveau-né)

Baby bottle - (Biberon)
Baby teeth - (Dent de lait)
Bacillus - (Bacillus, bactérie)
Back - (Dos)
Back - (Dos)
Back of the feet - (Dos du pied)
Back of the hand - (Dos de la main)
Back of, the; behind, the - (Partie arrière)
Backside; reverse side - (Face antérieure)
Bacteremia - (Bactériémie)
Bacteremic - (Bactériémique)
Bacteria - (Bactérie)
bacteria - (bactéries)
Bacteria, fecal coliform - (Bactérie fécale coliforme)
Bacterial - (Bactérien)
Bactericidal - (Bactericide, germicide)
Bacteriologist - (Bactériologiste)
Bacteriostatic - (Bactériostatique)
Bacteriuria - (Bactérionurie)
Bad - (Mal)
Bad/sick - (Mauvais)
Balance - (Balance)
Balanitis - (Balanite)
Balanoposthitis - (Balanopostite)
Baldness - (Calvitie)
Balsamic - (Pommade)

Bandage - (Bandage)
Bandage - (Bandage)
Bandage, to - (Mettre un bandage)
Band-aid - (Pansement adhésif)
Barbiturate - (Barbiturique)
Barefoot - (Pieds nus)
Barium Sulfate - (Sulfate de Barium)
Baroreceptor - (Barorécepteur)
Barr corpuscle - (Corps de Barr)
Barr corpuscle; Barr body - (Corpuscule de Barr)
Barrier - (Barrière)
Basal - (Basal)
Base - (Base)
Basophilic - (Basophile)
Bath - (Bain)
Bathe, to - (Baigner)
Be, to - (Etre)
Beat (as in heart beat) - (Battement)
Beat, rythmic cardiac - (Battement cardiaque rythmique)
Bed - (Lit)
Bed rest - (Rester au lit)
Begining - (Commencement, début)
Beginning - (Début)
Behavior - (Comportement)
Behind - (Derrière)
Belladonna - (Belladone)

Belly - (Ventre)
Belly button - (Nombril)
Benefit - (Bénéfice)
Benign - (Bénin)
Bent inward - (Varus)
Benzocaine - (Benzocaïne)
Beriberi - (Béribéri)
berseem - (berseem)
Better than - (Mieux, meilleur)
Bibliography - (Bibliographie)
Biceps - (Biceps)
Bicuspid - (Bicuspid)
Bifocals - (Lunettes bifocales)
Big toe - (Gros orteil)
Bigamy - (Bigamie)
Bigger - (Plus grand)
Bilateral - (Bilatéral (e))
Bile - (Bile)
bile - (même)
bile duct - (Tube)
Biliary - (Biliaire)
Bilirubin - (Bilirubine)
Bilirubinemia - (Bilirubinémie)
Bimanual - (Bimanuel)
Bioavailability - (Biodisponibilité)
Biochemistry - (Biochimie)
Biocompatible - (Biocompatibilité)
Biodegradable - (Biodégradation)
Bioequivalent - (Bioéquivalent)
Biology - (Biologie)
Biopsy - (Biopsie)
Biostatistic - (Biostatistique)
Biosyntesis - (Biosynthèse)

Biotin - (Biotine)
Biotype - (Biotype)
Biped - (Bipède)
birth - (Accouchement)
Birth - (Mise au monde, accoucher)
Birth - (Naissance)
Birth certificate - (Certificat de naissance, actede naissance)
Birth defect - (Défaut de naissance)
Birth rate - (Natalité)
Birth rate - (Taux de natalité)
Birth, home - (Accouchement à domicile)
Birth, premature - (Naissance prématurée)
Birthday - (Anniversaire)
Birthmark; mole - (Nævus)
Bisexual - (Bisexuel)
Bite - (Morsure)
Bite (e.g. of insect) - (Piqûre)
Bite, mosquito - (Piqûre de moustique)
Bitter - (Amer(ère))
Black - (Noir, noire)
Bladder - (Vessie)
bladder - (La vessie)
Bleed, to - (Saigner)
Bleed, to - (Saigner)
Bleeding - (Saignée)
Bleeding, Gastrointestinal - (Saignée gastro-intestinale)
Bleeding; bloody - (Saignement)

Blepharitis - (Blépharite)
Blepharo-conjuntivitis - (Blépharo-conjonctivite)
Blepharoplegia - (Blépharoplégie)
Blepharoptosis - (Blépharoptose)
Blepharospasm - (Blépharospame)
Blind - (Aveugle)
Blindness - (Cecité)
Blink - (Clignement des yeux)
blister - (blister)
Bloat - (Tympanite)
bloat - (Maladie)
Bloated - (Météorisme)
Block, to; prevent, to - (Empêcher)
Blockade (as in anesthetic regional block) - (Blocus)
Blood - (Sang)
Blood alcohol - (Alcoolémie)
Blood analysis - (Analyse du sang)
Blood analysis - (Analyse sanguin)
Blood Biometric - (Biométrie hématique)
blood cell - (globules)
Blood clot - (Caillot de sang)
Blood culture - (Hémoculture)
Blood flow - (Flux sanguin)
Blood irrigation - (Irrigation sanguine)
blood pressure - (La pression

artérielle)
Blood products - (Dérivés du sang)
blood sample - (échantillon de sang)
blood smear - (frottis de sang)
Blood supply - (Banque de sang)
Blood type - (Groupe sanguin)
Blood volume - (Volume sanguin)
Blood, Occult - (Sang caché)
Blood, Venous - (Sang veineux)
Bloodbank - (Banque de sang)
Bloody - (Ensanglanté(e))
Bloody Sputum - (Crachat sanguinolente)
Blow - (Coup)
blow - (Souffle)
blowfly - (blowfly)
Blue - (Bleu)
Body - (Corps)
Body fluid; humor; mood - (Humeur)
Boil, to - (Bouillir)
Boiled water - (Eau bouillie)
Bone - (Os)
Bone - (Osseux (se))
Born, to be - (Naître)
Bottle - (Bouteille)
Botulism - (Botulisme)
Bowlegged - (Cagneux)
Bradycardia - (Bradycardie)
Bradypnea - (Bradypnée)

Brain - (Cerveau)
bran - (son)
Branch - (Branche)
Bravery - (Valeur, courage)
Bread - (Pain)
Break, to - (Casser, briser)
Break, to - (Casser, se casser)
Breast - (Sein)
Breast milk; mother's milk - (Lait de mère)
Breastfeed - (Allaiter)
Breastfeeding - (Allaitement maternel)
Breath, bad - (Mauvaise haleine)
Breath; strength - (Haleine)
Breathe, to - (Respirer)
Broken - (Brisé(e), cassé(e))
Broken - (Cassé (e))
Bronchial aspiration - (Broncho-aspiration)
Bronchiectasis - (Bronchectasie)
Bronchiolitis - (Bronchite)
Bronchiotomy - (Bronchotomie)
Bronchodilator - (Bronchodilatateur)
Bronchopneumonia - (Broncho pneumonie)
Bronchopulmonary - (Bronchopulmonaire)
Bronchorrhea - (Bronchorrhée)
Bronchoscope - (Broncoscopie)

bronchus - (bronche)
Brother / sister - (Frère/ Sœur)
Brown - (Marron)
Brucellosis - (Brucellose)
Bruise - (Contusion)
Bruise; purple - (Bleu)
Brush - (Brosse)
Bruxism - (Bruxomanie)
Buccal - (Buccal)
Bulge; make bulge, to - (Bomber)
Bulky; swollen - (Volumineux)
Bunion - (Oignon)
burdizzo   - (Burdizzo outil pour la castration des animaux (p.11))
Burned - (Brûlé (e))
Burning sensation - (Ardeur)
Burns - (Brûlures)
Bursitis - (Bursite)
But - (Mais)
Butter - (Beurre)
Buttock (butt) - (Fesse)
Buzzing - (Bourdonnement)

~ C ~

Cachexia - (Cachexie)
Cadaver - (Cadavre)
caecum   - (caecum)
Calamine - (Calamine)
Calcemia - (Calcémie)
Calcification - (Calcification)

Calcium - (Calcium)
Calciuria - (Taux de calcium dans l'urine)
Calf (of leg) - (Mollet)
Callus; corn - (Cor, callosité)
Calm - (Tranquille)
Calm, to - (Calmer)
Calming; that which calms - (Calmant)
Calorie - (Calorie)
Canal - (Canal)
Cancer - (Cancer)
Cancerous - (Cancéreux)
Candida - (Candida)
Candidiasis - (Candidiase)
Candidiasis of the skin - (Dermo candidiase)
Cane - (Canne, bâton)
Canine tooth - (Canin)
Canine tooth - (Canine)
Cannula - (Canule)
Cap - (Couvercle, bouchon)
Capable - (Capable)
Capacity - (Capacité)
Capsule - (Capsule)
Carbohydrate - (Carbohydrate)
Carbon - (Charbon)
Carbonic acid - (Acide carbonique)
Carbuncle - (Furoncle)
Carcinogen - (Cancérigène)
Carcinogen - (Carcinogène)
Carcinoma - (Carcinome)
Cardiac - (Cardia)

Cardiac - (Cardiaque)
Cardiac massage - (Massage cardiaque)
Cardiac output - (Usure cardiaque)
Cardialgia - (Cardialgie)
Cardinal - (Cardinal)
Cardiogram - (Cardiogramme)
Cardiograph - (Cardiographie)
Cardiologist - (Cardiologue)
Cardiology - (Cardiologie)
Cardiomegaly - (Cardiomégalie)
Cardiomegaly - (Cardiomégalie)
Cardiomyopathy - (Cardiomyopathie)
Cardiopulmonary - (Cardio-pulmonaire)
Cardiotonic - (Cardiotonique)
Cardiovascular - (Cardiovasculaire)
Cardioverson - (Cardioversion)
Care - (Attention)
Care - (Soin)
Care for a prolonged life - (Soin pour prolonger la vie)
Care for unweaned babies - (Soin pendant l'allaitement,soin du nourrison)
Care for, to - (Soigner)
Care of convalescent - (Soin du convalescent)
Carotene - (Carotène)
Carotenemia - (Carotinémie)
Carotid - (Carotide)

Carpus - (Carpe)
Carrier - (Porteur)
carrier - (support)
Cartilage - (Cartilage)
Case - (Cas)
Case index - (Cas index)
Casket - (Cercueil)
Castrate, to - (Châtrer)
Castrated - (Châtré)
Catabolism - (Catabolisme)
Catalepsy - (Catalepsie)
Catalyze, to - (Cataliser)
Cataplasm - (Cataplasme)
Cataract - (Cataracte)
Catarrhal - (Catarrhal)
Catecholamine - (Catécholamine)
Catheter - (Cathéter)
Catheterize, to - (Mettre un cathéter, cathétériser)
Caudal; volume of flow - (Caudal)
Causal - (Causal)
Causal agent - (Agent causal)
Cause - (Cause)
Cause, to - (Occasionner)
cauterise - (cautériser)
Cave - (Cave)
Cavern - (Caverne)
Cavernous body of the penis - (Corps caverneux du pénis)
Cavities (dental) - (Carie dentaire)
Cavity - (Antre, cavité organique)
Cavity - (Cavité)

Cecum - (Caecum)
Celiac - (Coeliaque)
Cell - (Cellule)
Cell count - (Recomptage de cellules)
Cellulitis - (Cellullite)
Census; count - (Recensement)
Center - (Centre)
Centigrade - (Centigrade)
Centimeter - (Centimètre)
Central - (Central)
Cephalexin - (Céphalexine)
Cephalia - (Céphalée)
Cephalic - (Céphalique)
Cephalosporin - (Céphalosporine)
Cerclage - (Cerclage)
Cerebellospinal - (Cervelet-spinal)
Cerebellum - (Cervelet)
Cerebral Cortex - (Cortex cérébral)
Cerebral embolism - (Embolie cérébrale)
Cerebral hemorrhage - (Hémorragie cérébrale)
Cerebrospinal - (Cérébro-spinal)
Cerebrospinal fluid - (Liquide cérébro-spinal)
Cerebrovascular - (Cérébrovasculaire)
Certificate - (Acte)
Certificate - (Certificat)

Certify a death, to - (Certifier une mort)
Cervical - (Cervical)
Cervicitis - (Cervicite)
Cervix - (Cervical, relatif au cou)
Cervix - (Col de l'utérus)
cervix - (col)
Cesarean - (Césarienne)
Chair - (Chaise)
Chair (armchair) - (Balançoire)
Chalazion - (Chalazion)
Chancre - (Chancre)
Change - (Change)
Channel, to - (Canaliser)
Channel; tract - (Voie)
Chapped lips - (Lèvres gercées)
Character - (Caractère)
Cheap - (Bon marché, pas cher)
Cheek - (Joue)
Cheek - (Joue)
Cheilitis - (Chéilite)
Cheilosis - (Cheilose)
Chemist - (Chimiste)
Chemistry - (Chimie)
Chemoprophylaxis - (Chimio prophylaxie)
Chemoreceptor - (Chimiorécepteur)
Chemotherapy - (Chimiothérapie)
Chest - (Buste)
Chest - (Poitrine)

Chew, to - (Mastiquer, mâcher)
Chewer - (Masticateur)
Chicken Pox - (Varicelle)
Chicken Pox - (Varicelle Zona)
Child - (Garçon / Fille)
Child abuse - (Abus sur des enfants)
Childcare - (Soin de l'enfant)
Childhood - (Enfance)
Children's; childhood - (Infantile)
Chin - (Menton)
Chin, tip of the - (Menton)
Chiropraxis; chiropractic - (Chiropraxie)
Chlamydia - (Chlamydia)
Chloasma - (Chloasme)
Chlorhydric acid - (Acide chlorhydrique)
Chloroquine - (Chloroquine)
Chlorpromazine - (Chlorpromazine)
Cholangitis - (Cholangite)
Cholecystitis - (Cholecystite)
Choledochus - (Cholédoque)
Cholelithiasis - (Cholélitiase)
Cholera - (Choléra)
Cholestasis - (Cholestase)
Cholesterol - (Cholestérol)
Choleystectomy - (Cholecystectomie)
Cholinergic - (Cholinergique)
Choluria - (Urine obscure)
Chorea - (Chorée)
Choriocarcinoma - (Carcinome du chorion)
Chorion; corium - (Chorion)
Chromatine - (Chromatine)
Chromosome - (Chromosome)
Chronic - (Chronique)
chronic disease - (maladies chroniques)
Chronic illness, person with a - (Mal en point, patraque)
Chronicity - (Chronicité)
Cigarette - (Cigarette)
Ciliary - (Ciller)
Circle - (Cercle)
Circulation - (Circulation)
Circumcision - (Circoncision)
Cirrhosis - (Cirrhose)
Clarification - (Éclaircissement)
Classification - (Classification)
Classroom - (Classe)
Claudication, intermittent - (Claudification intermittente)
Clavicle - (Clavicule)
Claw hand - (Doigts en griffes)
Clean - (Propre)
Clean up - (Faire sa toilette)
Clear; Okay - (Clair(e))
Climate - (Climat)
Clinic - (Clinique)
Clinical - (Clinique)
Clinical history - (Dossier médical)
Clitoris - (Clitoris)
Clone - (Clone)
Cloning - (Clonage)

Close, to - (Fermer)
Closed - (Fermé (e))
clot - (caillot)
Clothing - (Linge)
Clouded - (Trouble)
clover - (trèfle)
Cluster; bunch - (Grappe)
CMV; Cytomegalovirus -
(CMV-cytomégalovirus)
Coagulation - (Coagulation)
Cocaine - (Cocaïne)
Coccyx - (Coccyx)
Coccyx - (Coccyx)
Codeine - (Codéine)
Coherent - (Cohérent)
Coitus - (Coït)
Cold - (Froid (e))
Cold, a - (Grippe, rhume)
Cold, to catch a - (Attraper
une grippe)
Cold, to catch a -
(S'enrhumer)
Cold; upper respiratory
infection - (Enrhumé)
Colectomy - (Colectomie)
Colic - (Colique)
colic - (coliques)
Colitis - (Colite)
Colitis, ulcerative - (Colite
ulcéreuse)
Collagenosis - (Collagénose)
Collapse - (Collapsus)
Collateral effect - (Effet
collatéral)
Colleague - (Collègue)

Collection; reception - (Attrait)
Collutorium - (Rince bouche,
bains de bouche, collutoire)
Collyrium - (Collyre)
Colon - (Colon)
Colonize - (Coloniser)
Colony - (Colonie)
Coloration - (Coloration)
Colorblind - (Daltonien)
Colostomy - (Colostomie)
Colostrum - (Colostrum)
colostrum - (colostrum)
Colposcopy - (Colposcopie)
Coma - (Coma)
Comatose - (Comateux(euse))
Combination - (Combinaison)
Commotion - (Commotion)
Communicate - (Se
communiquer)
Community - (Communauté)
Companion -
(Accompagnateur)
Compatible - (Compatible)
Compensate - (Compenser)
compensate - (compenser)
Complaint - (Plainte)
Complement - (Complément)
Complexion - (Peau (couleur))
Complexion; skin - (Peau de
visage)
Complicated - (Compliqué)
Complicated pregnancy -
(Grossesse compliquée)
Complication - (Complication)
Comprehend - (Comprendre)

Compress - (Compresse)
Computed Tomography (CT) -
(Tomographie Axial par
ordinateur (CAT scan))
Computer - (Ordinateur)
Computer - (Ordinateur)
Concentration -
(Concentration)
Concept - (Concept)
Conception - (Conception)
condition - (Affection)
Condition - (Condition)
Condom - (Condom)
Condom - (Préservatif)
Conduction - (Conduction)
Conduit - (Conduit)
Condyle - (Condyle)
Condyloma - (Condylome)
Conference - (Conférence)
Confidence - (Confiance)
Confidential - (Confidentiel)
Confinement of mental patient
- (Isolement du malade
mental)
Confirm, to - (Confirmer)
Confirmed diagnosis -
(Diagnostic confirmé)
Confuse - (Confus(e))
Confusion - (Confusion)
Congenital - (Congénital (e))
Congenital anomaly -
(Anomalie congénitale)
Congestion - (Congestion)
conjunctiva - (peau
conjonctive)
Conjunctive - (Conjonctive)

Conjunctivitis - (Conjonctivite)
Connection - (Connection)
Consanguinity -
(Consanguinité)
Conscience - (Conscience)
Conscious - (Conscient)
Conscious - (Conscient)
Conserve - (Conserver)
Constipated - (Constipé (e))
Constipated - (Constipé(e))
Constipation - (Constipation)
Constipation - (Constipation)
Constitution - (Constitution)
Consume - (Consommer)
Consumption; Tuberculosis -
(Tuberculose)
Consumptive - (Phtisique,
tuberculeux)
Contact - (Contact)
Contagion - (Contagion)
Contagious - (Contagieux)
contaminate - (contaminer)
Contamination; pollution -
(Contamination)
Content - (Contenu)
Continue - (Poursuivre)
Contraception -
(Contraception)
Contraceptive - (Contraceptif)
Contraceptive -
(Contraception)
Contraceptive -
(Contraception)
Contracted - (Contracté(e))
Contractile - (Contractile)
Contraction - (Contraction)

Contracture - (Contracture)
Contraindication - (Contre-indication)
Control - (Contrôler)
Control of drugs and narcotics - (Contrôle des médicaments et narcotiques)
Control of medicine; drugs - (Contrôle des médicaments)
Control of plagues - (Contrôle de fléaux)
Control of transmitable diseases - (Contrôle des maladies transmissibles)
Contusion - (Contusion)
Convalescence - (Convalescence)
Convulsion - (Convulsion)
convulsions - (convulsions)
Cooling - (Refroidissement)
Cooperate - (Coopérer)
Coordinate - (Coordonner)
Coproculture - (Coproculture)
Copulation - (Copule)
Cord - (Corde)
Cornea - (Cornée)
cornea - (cornée)
Coronary - (Coronarien)
Coronary arteries - (Artères coronaires)
Corporal - (Corporel)
Corpus callosum - (Callosité)
Corpus luteum - (Corps jaune(corpus luteum))
Correct - (Correct (e))

Correct diagnosis - (Bon diagnostic)
Cortex - (Cortex)
Corticosteroids - (Corticostéroïdes)
Corticotropin - (Corticotrophine)
Cortisol - (Cortisol, hydro-cortisone)
Cotton - (Coton)
Cough - (Toux)
Coughing - (Tousser)
Coughing spell - (Quinte de toux)
Courage; state of mind - (Courage)
Cover - (Abriter)
Cover - (Couvrir)
Cover - (Couvrir)
Coverage - (Couverture)
Coxalgia - (Coxalgie)
Coxofemoral - (Coxofémoral)
Cradle - (Berceau)
Cramp - (Crampe)
Cramps - (Crampes)
Cranial - (Crânien)
Cranium - (Crâne)
Crash - (Accident)
Crash - (choc)
Cream - (Crème)
Creatinine - (Créatinine)
Cretinism, hypothyroidism - (Crétinisme)
Crisis - (Crise)
Criteria - (Critère)

crop   - (culture)
Crutches - (Béquilles)
Cry, to - (Pleurer)
Cryosurgery - (Cryochirurgie)
Cryptorchidy - (Cryptorchidie)
Crystalization - (Cristalisation)
Cubital - (Cubital)
Curable - (Guérissable)
Cure by resting - (Cure de repos)
Cure, to - (Soigner)
Cure; priest (as one curing souls) - (Cure)
Curettage - (Curetage)
Curettage - (Curetage, avortement)
Curettage; scrape; scraped - (Râpé)
Curve - (Courbe)
Custom; habit - (Habitude)
Cut (noun) - (Coupe)
Cut (verb) - (Couper)
Cyanosis - (Cyanose)
Cyanotic - (Cyanosé)
Cyclical - (Ciclique)
Cyclothymia - (Cyclotimie)
Cyst - (Kyste)
cyst   - (kyste)
Cystadenoma - (Cystadenome)
Cystic - (Kystique)
Cystic fibrosis - (Fibrose kystique)
Cystitis - (Cystite)
Cystoscopy - (Cystoscopie)
Cytology - (Cytologie)

Cytolysis - (Cytolyse)
Cytopenia - (Cytopénie)
Cytoplasm - (Cytoplasme)
Cytotoxic - (Cytotoxique)

~ D ~

Dacryocystitis - (Dacryocystite)
Damage, to; injure - (Blesser, faire mal)
Damage; injury - (Mal)
Dangerous - (Dangereux)
Dark - (Foncé (e))
Database - (Base de données)
Date - (Date)
Daughter - (Fille)
Day - (Jour)
Days of rest - (Jours de repos)
Days on bed rest - (Jours au lit)
Dead; cadaver - (Mort, cadavre)
Deaf - (Sourd, sourde)
Deaf-Mute - (Sourd-muet)
Deafness - (Surdité)
Dean - (Doyen)
Death - (Mort, décès)
Death certificate - (Certificat de décès)
Death certificate - (Certificat de décès)
Death encephalic; brain death - (Mort encéphalique)
Death, sudden; sudden infant

death syndrome - (Mort subite)
Debridement - (Débridement)
Decerebrate - (Décérébration)
Decidual - (Déciduale)
Deciliter - (Décilitre)
Decision - (Décision)
Decompose - (Décomposer)
Decomposition - (Décomposition)
Decongest, to - (Décongestionner)
Decongestant - (Décongestionnant)
Decongestion - (Décongestion)
Decontamination - (Décontamination)
Decortication - (Décortication)
Decrease - (Décroître)
Decrease - (Diminution, baisse)
Deep breath - (Respiration profonde)
Defecate, to - (Déféquer)
Defecation; bowel movement - (Défécation)
Defect; flaw - (Défaut)
Defense - (Défense)
Defer - (Différer)
Deferent duct - (Canal déférent)
Defibrillation - (Défibrillation)
Defibrillator - (Défibrillateur)
Deficiency - (Déficience)

Deficit - (Déficit)
Defloration - (Défloration)
Deformation - (Déformation)
Degeneration - (Dégénérescence)
Degenerative - (Dégénératif (ve))
Degradation - (Dégradation)
Degree - (Degré)
Dehiscence - (Déhiscence)
Dehydrated - (Déshydraté)
Dehydration - (Déshydratation)
dehydration - (déshydratation)
Delay; lag - (Retard)
Delay; retardation - (Retard)
Delayed effects - (Effets tardifs)
Delirium - (Délire)
Delivery - (Accouchement)
Delivery; breech - (Présentation de siège)
Delouse - (Epouiller)
Deltoids - (Deltoïdes)
Dementia - (Démence)
Demography - (Démographie)
Demonstration; sign - (Démonstration)
Demyelination - (Démyélinisation)
Dendrite - (Dendrite)
Dengue - (Dengue)
Denomination - (Dénomination)

Dental assistance - (Assistance dentaire)
Dental care, preventive - (Odontologie préventive)
Dentist - (Dentiste)
Dentition - (Dentition)
Denture - (Dentition)
Deontology - (Déontologie)
Deoxyribonucleic acid - (Acide désoxirhydrique)
Department - (Département)
Dependency - (Dépendance)
Dependent - (Dépendant)
Depersonalization - (Dépersonnalisation)
Depletion - (Déplétion)
Depressed - (Abattu)
Depressed - (Découragé, déprimé)
Depth - (Profondeur)
Derived - (Dérivé(e))
Dermatitis - (Dermatite)
Dermatological - (Dermatologique)
Dermatologist - (Dermatologue)
Dermatology - (Dermatologie)
Dermatomycoses - (Dermatomycose)
Dermatosis - (Dermatose)
Descendence - (Descendance)
Desensitize - (Désensibilisation)
Desquamation - (Desquamation)
Detect, to - (Détecter)

Detection - (Détection)
Deteriorate - (Détériorer)
Detoxification - (Désintoxication)
Develop - (Développer)
Development - (Développement)
Developmental delay; mental retardation - (Retard mental)
Device - (Dispositif)
Dexamethasone - (Dexaméthasone)
Dextrocardia - (Dextrocardie)
Dextrose - (Dextrose)
Diabetes - (Diabète)
Diabetes Mellitus - (Diabète mellitus)
Diabetic - (Diabétique)
Diabetic acidosis - (Acidose diabétique)
Diagnose - (Diagnostiquer)
Diagnostic - (Diagnostic)
Diaper - (Couche)
Diaphoresis, sweat - (Diaphorèse)
Diaphragm - (Diaphragme)
Diaphysis, shaft of a bone - (Diaphyse)
Diarrhea - (Diarrhée)
diarrhoea - (diarrhée)
Diastole - (Diastole)
Diastolic - (Diastolique)
Diathesis - (Diathèse)
Diazepam - (Valium, diazépam)
Dichotomy - (Dichotomie)

Dictionary - (Dictionnaire)
Die, to - (Mourir)
Die, to; pass away, to -
(Mourir, décéder)
Diencephalon - (Diencéphale)
Diet - (Alimentation)
Diet - (Diète)
Dietary supplement -
(Alimentation supplémentaire)
Differentiation -
(Différenciation)
Diffuse, to; spread out, to -
(Diffuser, reprendre)
Diffuse; unclear - (Diffuse)
Digest - (Digérer)
Digestion - (Digestion)
digestion - (digestion)
Digestive - (Digestif (ive))
Digestive system - (Appareil
digestif)
Digital - (Digital)
Digitalization - (Digitalisation)
Digitoxin - (Digitoxine)
Dilatation - (Dilatation)
Dilution - (Dilution)
Diminish; reduce - (Diminuer)
Diphtheria - (Diphtérie)
Diplagia - (Paralysé des deux
côtés)
Diplococcus - (Diplocoque)
Diplodia - (Champion qui
pousse sur lesplantes)
Diplophonia - (Diplophonie)
Diplopia - (Diplopie)
Dipsomania - (Dipsomanie)

Dipstick - (Bande réactive)
Direct - (Direct)
Dirty - (Sale)
Disabilities, person with -
(Handicapé)
Disability - (Incapacité)
Disabled - (Incapable)
Disabled; handicapped -
(Handicapé)
Disarticulate - (Désarticuler)
Disasters - (Désastres)
discharge - (décharger)
Discharge; drainage; flow -
(Flux)
Discoid - (Discoïde)
Discomfort; nuisance - (Gène,
dérangement)
Discover - (Découvrir)
Discussion - (Discussion)
disease - (Affection)
disease - (maladie)
Disease outbreak - (Premiers
signes d'une épidémie)
Disgust; nausea - (Dégoût)
Disinfect, to - (Désinfecter)
Disinfectant - (Désinfectant)
Disinfection - (Désinfection)
Dislocated - (Déboîter)
Dislocation - (Débôitement)
Dislocation - (Désajustement)
Dislocation - (Luxation)
dislocation - (dislocation)
Disorder - (Trouble)
Disoriented - (Désorienté)
Dispareunia; painful sex -

(Dyspareunie)
Dispensary - (Dispensaire)
Dispersion - (Dispersion)
Displacement - (Déplacement)
Disposable - (Jetable)
Disposition - (Disposition)
Disseminated - (Disséminé(e))
Dissociation - (Dissociation)
Dissolution - (Dissolution)
Distal - (Distal)
Distention - (Distension)
Distill - (Suinter, distiller)
Distilled water - (Eau distillée)
Distortion - (Entorse,
distorsion)
Distribute, to; share, to -
(Distribuer, partager)
Distribution - (Distribution)
Diuresis - (Diurèse)
Diuretic - (Diurétique)
Diverticulitis - (Diverticulite)
Diverticulosis - (Diverticulose)
Diverticulum - (Diverticule)
Dizziness - (Perte de
conscience)
Do, to; make, to - (Faire)
Doctor - (Docteur)
Doctor - (Médecin)
Doctor (female) - (Docteure)
Doctor, family - (Médecin de
famille)
Doctor's appointment -
(Consultation)
Doctor's orders - (Prescription
facultative)
Documents - (Documents)

Dominance - (Domination,
Contrôle)
Dominant - (Dominant)
Dominant characteristic -
(Héritage dominant)
Done; made; fact; data -
(Fait)
Donor - (Donneur)
Dorsal - (Dorsal)
Dosage - (Dose)
Dose - (Dose)
Dotted; stippled; sutured -
(Pointillé)
Doubt - (Doute)
Doxycycline - (Doxycycline)
Drain - (Drainer)
Drainage - (Drainage)
Dressed - (Robe, habit)
Dressing - (Pansement)
Drink, to - (Boire)
Drinker - (Ivrogne)
Drinking water - (Eau potable)
Drooling - (Hypersalivation)
Drop; drip - (Goutte)
Drown, to; choke, to - (Se
noyer, s'étouffer)
Drowning - (Étouffement,
noyade)
Drowsy - (Endormi(e))
Drug abuse - (Abus de
drogues)
Drug addict - (Drogué(e))
Drug addiction - (toxicomanie)
Drug dependency -
(Toxicomane)
Drug(s) - (Drogue(s))

Drugstore; Pharmacy - (Pharmacie)
Drunk - (Ivrogne, soulard)
Dry - (Sec, sèche)
dry birth - (Accouchement á sec)
Dry, to - (Sécher)
Duct - (Conduit)
Duodenitis - (Duodénite)
Duodenoscopy - (Duodénoscopie)
Duodenum - (Duodénum)
During - (Durant)
Dying person - (Mourant(e))
Dysarthria - (Dysarthrie)
Dyscrasia - (Dyscrasie)
Dysentery - (Dysenterie)
Dysesthesia - (Dysesthésie)
Dysfunction - (Dysfonctionnement)
Dysgenesis - (Dysgénésie)
Dyskinesia - (Dyskinésie)
Dysmenorrhea - (Dysménorrhée)
Dyspepsia - (Dyspepsie)
Dysphagia - (Dysphagie)
Dysphonia - (Dysphonie)
Dysplasia - (Dysplasie)
Dyspnea - (Dyspnée)
Dyspneic - (Dyspnéique)
Dystocia - (Dystocie)
Dystrophy - (Dystrophie)
Dysuria - (Dysurie)

~ E ~

Ear - (Oreille)
Ear (outer) - (Oreille)
Ear and throat, study of - (Otolaryngologie)
Ear nose & throat, Study of; ENT - (Oto- rhino- laryngologie)
Earache - (Otalgie)
Eardrum; Tympanum - (Tympan)
Ears, ringing in the - (Bourdonnement des oreilles)
Earwax - (Cérumen)
Easy - (Facile)
Eat - (Manger)
Ecchymosis; bruise - (Ecchymose)
Echo - (Echo)
Echocardiography - (Echocardiographie)
Echography - (Echographie)
Eclampsia - (Eclampsie)
Economy - (Economie)
Ectasia - (Ectasie)
Ectopic pregnancy - (Grossesse ectopique)
Ectopy - (Ectopie)
Eczema - (Eczéma)
Edema - (Oedème)
Edematous - (Oedémateux (euse))
Education - (Education)

Effect - (Effet)
Effective - (Efficace)
Effort - (Effort)
Effusion - (Effusion)
Egg - (Oeuf)
Eighth - (Huitième)
Ejaculate - (Éjaculer)
Ejaculation - (Éjaculation)
Elastic - (Élastique)
Elbow - (Coude)
Electricity - (Electricité)
Electrocardiogram -
(Electrocardiogramme)
Electroencephalogram; EEG -
(ElectroencéphalogrammeEEG)
Electrolyte - (Electrolyte)
Electrolytic imbalance -
(Déséquilibre électrolytique)
Electromyogram; EMG -
(Electromyogramme EMG)
Element - (Elément)
Elephantiasis - (Éléphantiasis)
Eliminate - (Eliminer)
Elimination - (Elimination)
Elixir - (Elixir)
Embolism - (Embolie)
Embolism - (Embolisme)
Embolus, emboli (pl) - (Piston)
Embryo - (Embryon)
Embryology - (Embryologie)
Emergencies - (Urgences)
Emergency - (Urgence)
Emergency care - (Soins
d'urgence)
Emergency department -
(Département des urgences)

Emergency medical team -
(Service d'Urgences)
Emetic - (Émétique)
Emollient - (Émollient)
Emotion - (Emotion)
Emphysema - (Emphysème)
Emphysematous -
(Emphysémateux)
Empty - (Vide)
Empyema - (Empyème)
Emulsion - (Emulsion)
Enanthem; rash on mucous
membranes - (Énanthème)
Encapsulated - (En capsule)
Encephalitis - (Encéphalite)
Encephalomyelitis -
(Encéphalomyélite)
Encephalopathy -
(Encéphalopathie)
Encephalus; brain -
(Encéphale)
Encopresis - (Encoprésie)
End - (Fin)
Endaortitis - (Endaortite)
Endarterectomy -
(Endartériectomie)
Endarteritis - (Endartérite)
Endemic - (Endémie)
Endemic - (Endémique)
Endocarditis - (Endocardite)
Endocarditis - (Qui souffre
d'endocardite)
Endocardium - (Endocarde)
Endocrine - (Endocrine)
Endocrine glands - (Glandes
endocrines)

Endocrinology - (Endocrinologie)
Endogenous - (Endogène)
Endometriosis - (Endométriose)
Endometritis - (Endométrite)
Endometrium - (Endomètre)
Endoscopy - (Endoscopie)
Endothelium - (Endothélium)
Endotoxic - (Endotoxique)
Endotoxin - (Endotoxine)
Endure, to - (Supporter)
Enema - (Enéma, lavement)
Enema - (Poire a' lavement)
Energy - (Energie)
Enlargement - (Agrandissement)
Enough - (Assez)
Enteritis - (Entérite)
enteritis - (entérite)
Enterobiasis - (Entérobiase)
Enterocolitis - (Entérocolite)
Enteropathy - (Entéropathie)
Enterorrhagia; intestinal hemorrhage - (Hémorragie intestinale)
Enterotoxin - (Entérotoxine)
Enterovirus - (Entérovirus)
Entrails; innards; bowels - (Viscères)
Entrance; entryway - (Porte d'entrée)
Enuresis - (Énurésie)
Environment - (Environnement)

Environment - (Environnement)
Environmental control - (Environnement contrôlé)
enzootic - (enzootique)
Eosinophilia - (Éosinophilie)
Eosinophilic - (Éosinophile)
Epicondylitis - (Épicondylite)
Epidemic - (Épidémie)
Epidemic - (Épidémique)
Epidemiology - (Épidémiologie)
Epidermic - (Épidermique)
Epidermis - (Épiderme)
Epididymo - (Épididyme)
Epidural - (Épidural)
Epigastralgia - (Épigastralgie)
Epigastrium - (Épigastre)
Epiglottis - (Épiglotte)
Epiglottitis - (Inflammation de l'épiglotte)
Epilepsy - (Épilepsie)
Epileptic - (Épileptique)
Epileptic seizure - (Crise épileptique)
Epiphysis - (Épiphyse)
Epiphysis, in relation to - (En relation avec l'épiphyse)
Episiotomy - (Épisiotomie)
Episode - (Épisode)
Epistaxis - (Épistaxis)
Epithelioma - (Épithélioma)
Epithelium - (Épithélium)
epizootic - (épizootie)
Equal - (Egal)

Equilibrium - (Équilibre)
Equivalent - (Équivalent)
eradicate - (éradiquer)
Erection - (Érection)
Ergotherapy - (Ergothérapie)
Error - (Erreur)
Eructation; Burp; Belch -
(Éructation, faire des rots)
Eruption - (Éruption)
Erysipelas - (Érysipèle)
Erythema - (Érythème)
Erythrocyte - (Érythrocyte)
Erythrocytopenia - (Manque d'
érythrocytes)
Erythropoiesis -
(Érythropoïèse)
Eschar; scab - (Escarre)
Escherichia coli - (Éscherichia
Coli)
Esophagus - (Oesophage)
Estrogen - (Estrogène)
Ethic - (Éthique)
Etiologic - (Étiologique)
Etiology - (Étiologie)
Euphoria - (Euphorie)
Evacuate - (Évacuer)
Evacuation - (Évacuation)
Evagination - (Évagination)
Evaluation - (Évaluation)
Event - (Évènement)
Evil eye - (Mauvais oeil)
Evolution - (Évolution)
Exacerbation - (Exacerbation)
Exacerbation; attack (of
disease) - (Tirer avec force)
Exam - (Examen)

Examination; recognition -
(Auscultation, examen)
Examine, to - (Examiner)
Examine, to; recognize, to -
(Examiner, ausculter)
Example - (Exemple)
Exanthema - (Exanthème)
Excessive - (Excessif (ive))
Exchange - (Echange)
Excipient - (Excipient,
substance)
Excitement - (Agitation)
Excitement; arousal -
(Excitation)
Excrement - (Excrément)
Excrescence; protuberance -
(Protubérance)
Excretion - (Excrétion)
Exfoliation - (Exfoliation)
Exhale - (Exhaler)
Exhausted - (Épuisé (e))
Exit - (Porte de sortie)
Exit - (Sortie)
Exocrine - (Exocrine)
Exocrine glands - (Glandes
exocrines)
Exogenous - (Exogène)
Exophthalmic goiter - (Goitre
exophtalmique)
Exophthalmos - (Exophtalmie)
Expand; dilate - (Dilater)
Expectorant - (Expectorant)
Expectoration -
(Expectoration)
Expel - (Expulser)
Expense - (Dépense)

Experience - (Expérience)
Experimental -
(Expérimental(e))
Expiration - (Expiration)
Expire - (Expirer)
Expire, to (medication) -
(Expirer, périmer)
Exploration - (Exploration)
Exposed - (Exposé)
Exposition - (Exposition)
Extension - (Extension)
Exterior - (Extérieur)
Exterminate - (Exterminer)
External - (Externe)
Externalize - (Extérioriser)
Extirpate; remove - (Extirper)
Extirpation; removal -
(Extirpation)
Extract, to - (Extraire)
Extraction - (Extraction)
Extraction, dental - (Extraction
dentaire)
Extrasystole - (Extrasystole)
Extrauterine - (Extra-utérin)
Extravaginal - (Hors du vagin,
extra-vaginal)
Extravasation - (Extravasation)
Extravascular -
(Extravasculaire)
Extravesical - (Hors de la
vessie)
Extreme - (Extrême)
Extrophy - (Exstrophie)
Exuded - (Prélèvement
d'exsude ou sécrétion suintant)

Eye - (Oeil, yeux(pl))
Eye adnexa - (Organes de
l'œil :sourcils, cils, paupières,
glandes lacrymales.)
Eye strain - (Vue fatiguée)
Eyebrow - (Sourci)
Eyedropper - (Compte
gouttes)
Eyelash - (Cil)
Eyelid - (Paupière)

~ F ~

Face - (Visage)
Face - (Visage)
Face down - (Sur le ventre, à
plat ventre)
Face up - (Sur le dos)
Facial - (Facial(e))
Facies - (Faciès)
Factor - (Facteur)
Facultative - (Facultatif (ive))
faeces - (excréments)
Failure - (Échec)
Failure - (Erreur, défaillance)
Faint - (Evanouissement)
Faint - (Evanouissement)
Faint; pass out, to - (Défaillir,
s'évanouir)
Fainted - (Qui a perdu
connaissance)
Falciform; sickle shaped -
(Falciforme)
Fall - (Chute)

false - (Faux)
False teeth - (Faux dents)
Family - (Famille)
Family composition - (Composition familiale)
Family Planning Center - (Centre de planification familiale)
Famine - (Famine)
Fascicle; bundle - (Faisceau)
Fasciculation; involuntary contraction of muscle fibers - (Fasciculation, contraction desfibres musculaires involontaire)
Fasciola hepatica; liver fluke - (Fasciole hépatique)
Fasciola; genus of flukes, a - (Fasciole)
Fast (go without eating) - (A jeun)
Fast (go without eating) - (Jeûne)
Fat - (Graisse)
Fat; obese - (Gros, grosse, obèse)
Fatal - (Fatal (e))
Father - (Père)
Father; dad; papa - (Papa)
Father-in-Law - (Beau père/ Belle mère)
Fatigue - (Fatigue)
Fatigue - (Fatigue)
fatigued - (Accablement)
Fatigued; tired - (Fatigué, suffoqué)

Fatty - (Adipose)
Fear - (Peur)
Febrile - (Fiévreux(se))
Febrile convulsion; seizure - (Convulsion fiévreuse)
Febrile, feverish - (Fiévreux(se))
Febrile; feverish - (Fébrile)
Fecal - (Fécal)
Fecal culture - (Culture fécale, culture deselles)
Fecal matter - (Matières fécales)
Fecaloma; tumor of impacted feces - (Fécalome)
Feces - (Fèces)
Feces; fecal matter; shit - (Caca, selles, fèces)
Feed, to - (Alimenter)
Feel - (Sentir)
Feel pain, to - (Faire mal)
Feeling - (Sentiment)
Female - (Genre féminin)
Feminine - (Féminin (e))
Femur - (Fémur)
Fertile - (Fertile)
Fertile; fecund - (Fécondité)
fertiliser - (engrais minéraux)
Fertility - (Fertilité)
Fertilization; fecundation - (Fécondation)
Fertilize, to; fecundate, to - (Féconder)
Fetal - (Fœtal)
Fetal development - (Développement fœtal)

Fetography; fetal radiograph - (Fœtographie, radiographie dufœtus)

Fetometry; estimation of fetal size - (Fœtométrie, mesure du fœtus)

Fetoprotein - (Fœtoprotéine)

Fetus - (Fœtus)

Fever - (Fièvre)

fever - (fièvre)

Fibrillation - (Fibrillation)

Fibrin - (Fibrine)

Fibrinogen - (Fibrinogène)

Fibrinolysis - (Fibrinolyse)

Fibrinopenia - (Fibrinopénie, manque defibrine)

Fibroma - (Fibrome)

Fibromyositis - (Fibromyosite)

Fibrosis - (Fibrose)

Fibula - (Fibule, agrafe, péroné)

Fibula - (Péroné)

Fifth - (Cinquième)

Filling - (Plombage)

Filter - (Filtre)

Filtration - (Filtration)

Finger - (Doigt)

Fingerprint - (Empreintes digitales)

Fingertip - (Jaune d'œuf, bout(doigt))

Fire - (Incendie)

First - (Premier, première)

First aid - (Premier soins)

First aid kit - (Trousse d'urgence)

Fissure - (Fissure)

Fist - (Poignet)

Fistula - (Fistule)

Fixation - (Fixation)

Fixed denture - (Dentition définitive)

Flaccid; limp - (Flasque)

Flatulence - (Flatulence)

Flea - (Pou)

Fleeting - (Fugace)

Flexion - (Flexion)

Flora - (Flore)

Flu; influenza - (Grippe, Rhume)

Fluctuate - (Fluctuer)

Fluid - (Fluide)

flukes - (douves)

Fly - (Mouche)

flystrike - (flystrike)

foetus - (foetus)

Fold (noun) - (Pli)

Folic acid - (Acide folique)

Follicle - (Follicule)

Folliculitis - (Folliculite)

Fomites - (Fomites)

Fontanel - (Fontanelle)

Food - (Aliments)

Food - (Nourriture)

food aid - (Aide alimentaire)

Food poisoning - (Intoxication alimentaire)

Food Preservation - (Conservation d'aliments)

Food supplement -

(Suppléments alimentaires)
Food supply - (Approvisionnement d'aliments)
Foot, human - (Pied)
Foot; paw - (Patte)
For - (Pour)
Foramen; orifice - (Foramen, orifice)
Forceps - (Forceps)
Forearm - (Avant bras)
Forehead - (Front)
Foreign body - (Corps étranger)
Forensic - (Médecin légiste)
Form; shape - (Forme)
Fossa - (Fosse)
Fraction; part - (Fraction)
Fracture - (Fracture)
Fracture, hairline - (Os cassé)
Fracture; tear; breakage - (Cassure)
Free - (Gratuit)
Fremitus - (Frémir)
Frequency; rate - (Fréquence)
Fresh water - (Eau douce, potable)
Frigidity - (Frigidité)
Frontal - (Frontal(e))
Full - (Plein (e))
Fulminant - (Fulminant (e))
Fulminant hepatitis - (Hépatite fulminante)
Fumigate, to - (Fumiger)
Fumigation - (Fumigation)
Function - (Fonction)

Fundus of the eye - (Fond d'œil)
Fundus; base; bottom - (Fond)
Fundus; base; bottom - (Fond)
Fungicide - (Fongicide)
Fungus - (Fongus)
Fungus - (Fongus, champignon)
fungus - (champignon)
Furuncle - (Furoncle)
Furuncle - (Furoncle)
Future - (Futur)

~ G ~

Gain weight - (Gagner du poids)
Gain weight, to - (Grossir, engraisser)
Galactorrhea - (Galacthorrée)
Gall Bladder - (Vésicule biliaire)
gall bladder - (vésicule biliaire)
Gamma globulin - (Gammaglobuline)
Ganglion - (Ganglion)
Ganglion - (Ganglion)
Gangrene - (Gangrène)
Gargle - (Gargarisme, faire des gargarismes)
Gasoline - (Gazoline, essence)

Gastralgia; stomach ache - (Gastralgie)
Gastric acid - (Acidité gastrique)
Gastric juice - (Suc gastrique)
Gastritis - (Gastrite)
Gastroduodenal - (Gastro-duodénal)
Gastroenteritis - (Gastro-entérite)
gastro-enteritis - (gastro-entérite)
Gastroenterocolitis - (Gastro-entérocolite)
Gastroesophageal - (Gastro-œesophage)
Gastrointestinal - (Gastro-intestinal)
Gastroscopy - (Gastroscopie)
Gauze - (Gaze)
Gender - (Genre)
Gene - (Gène)
General - (Général)
Genesis; origin - (Genèse)
Genetic - (Génétique)
Genetic Counseling - (Conseil génétique)
Genetic disease - (Maladie génétique)
Genital - (Génital)
Genital herpes - (Herpès génital)
Genitalia, female - (Partie)
Genitals - (Génitaux)
Genome - (Génome)

Genotype - (Génotype)
Gentamycin - (Gentamicine)
Geriatric - (Gériatrique)
Geriatrics - (Gériatrie)
Germ - (Germe)
Germicide - (Germicide)
Gestation - (Gestation, grossesse)
Gestosis - (Gestose)
Get sick, to - (Tomber malade)
Get up, to; stand, to - (Se lever)
Giardia - (Giardia)
Giardiasis - (Giardiase, lambiose)
Gingiva; gums - (Gencive)
Gingivitis - (Gingivite)
Gingivorrhagia - (Gingivorragie)
Give - (Donner)
Give birth, to - (Accoucher)
gizzard - (gésier)
Gland - (Glande)
Gland - (Glande)
gland - (glande)
Glasses; eyeglasses - (Lunettes)
Glasses; eyeglasses - (Lunettes)
Glaucoma - (Glaucome)
Glomerular - (Glomérulaire)
Glomerulonephritis - (Glomérulonéphrite)
Glossalgia - (Glossalgie)
Glossitis - (Glossite)

Glottis - (Glotte)
Glove - (Gant)
Glucocorticoid -
(Glucocorticoïde)
Glucose - (Glucose)
Glucose levels - (Taux de
glucose)
Glucoside - (Glucoside)
Gluteus; buttock - (Fesse)
Glycemia - (Glycémie)
Glycemia - (Glycémie)
Glycogen - (Glycogène)
Glycopenia - (Glucopénie)
Glycosuria - (Glucourie)
go without eating - (A jeun)
Goal; aim - (But)
Goiter - (Goitre)
Gonad - (Gonade)
Gonadal - (Gonadique)
Gonadotropin -
(Gonadotrophine)
Gonorrhea - (Blennorragie)
Gonorrhea - (Gonorrhée)
Good - (Bien)
Good - (Bon/Bonne)
Good practice - (Bonne
practique)
Good visibility, to have - (Avoir
une bonne vue)
Graft - (Greffe)
Gram - (Gramme)
Gram - (Gramme)
Gram negative - (Gram-
négatif)
Gram positive - (Gram-positif)
Grandchild - (Petit fils/ Petite
fille)
Grandfather - (Grand-père,
grand- mère)
Granule - (Granule)
Granulocytopenia -
(Granulocytopénie)
Great Grandfather / Great
Grandmother - (Arrière grand-
père /Arrièregrand-mère)
Great Grandson / Great
Grandmother - (Arrière petit
fils /Arrière petitefille)
Green - (Vert)
Greet, to - (Saluer)
Grey - (Gris)
grief - (Affliction)
Grinding one's teeth; bruxism
- (Grincement des dents,
bruxisme)
Groan, to; complain, to - (Se
plaindre)
Groan; moan - (Plainte)
Groin - (Aine)
Group; type - (Groupe)
Grow, to - (Grandir, croître)
Growth - (Croissance)
Gum - (Gencive)
Gunshot wound - (Blessé par
balle)
Gynecologist - (Gynécologue)
Gynecology - (Gynécologie)
Gynecomastia -
(Gynécomastie)

~ H ~

Habit - (Habitude)
Habitual - (Habituel)
haemorrhage - (hémorragie)
Hair - (Cheveux)
Hair - (Poil, cheveu)
Hair on the body, face -
(Duvet)
Half - (Moitié)
Halitosis - (Halitose)
Hallucination - (Hallucination)
Hand - (Main)
Hand washing - (Lavage des
mains)
Happen, to - (Arriver)
Hard - (Dur(e))
Harmful - (Nocif)
Head - (Tête)
Head - (Tête)
Headache - (Mal de tête)
Heal, to - (Guérir)
Healing, to speed the process
of - (Accélérer la guérison)
Health - (Santé)
Health - (Service sanitaire)
Health administration -
(Administration sanitaire)
Health Center - (Centre de
santé)
Health certificate - (Certificat
de santé)
Health education - (Education
sanitaire)

Health form - (Feuille de route
clinique)
Health infrastructure -
(Infrastructure sanitaire)
Health personnel - (Personnel
de la santé)
Health promotion campaign -
(Campagne de promotion
desanté)
Health services administration
- (Administration des services
de santé)
Health standards - (Niveaux
d´attention de santé)
Health units - (Unités de
santé)
Health, environmental -
(Santé environnementale)
Health, maternal-child -
(Santé de la mère et du
nouveau-né)
Health, mental - (Santé
mentale)
Health, oral - (Santé buccale)
Health, public - (Santé
publique)
Healthy - (Sain (e), en bonne
santé)
Healthy (sound) - (Sain)
Healthy food - (Nourriture
saine)
Healthy life - (Vie saine)
Healthy person - (Personne
saine)
Hear, to - (Entendre)

Hearing - (Audition)
Hearing aid; auditory
apparatus - (Appareil
acoustique)
Heart - (Cœur)
Heart attack - (Crise
cardiaque)
Heart attack - (Crise
cardiaque)
Heart failure - (Asystolie)
Heart failure - (Insuffisance
cardiaque)
Heart noise - (Bruit cardiaque)
Heart rate - (Fréquence
cardiaque)
heartburn - (Acidité)
Heartburn - (Brûlure
d'estomac)
Heat - (Chaleur)
heat - (la chaleur)
Heavy - (Lourd (e))
Heel - (Talon)
Heel, Achilles - (Talon
d'Achille)
Height - (Hauteur)
helminths - (helminthes)
Help - (Soins, aide)
Help; aid; assistance - (Appui)
Hematemesis; vomiting blood
- (Hématémèse)
Hematocolpos; retained
menstruation -
(Haematocolpos)
Hematologic -
(Hématologique)
Hematoma - (Hématome)

Hematopoiesis -
(Hématopoïèse)
Hematuria; blood in the urine
- (Hématurie)
Hemiatrophy; atrophy of half -
(Hémiatrophie)
Hemicrania - (Hémicrânie)
Hemiparesis - (Hémiparésie)
Hemiplegia - (Hémiplégie)
Hemiplegic - (Hémiplégique)
Hemisphere - (Hémisphère)
Hemithorax - (Hémithorax)
Hemoconcentration - (Hémo-
concentration)
Hemodialysis - (Hémodialyse)
Hemoglobin - (Hémoglobine)
Hemoglobinopathy -
(Hémoglobinopathie)
Hemogram - (Hémogramme)
Hemolysis - (Hémolyse)
Hemophilia - (Hémophilie)
Hemoptysis - (Hémoptysie)
Hemorrhage - (Hémorragie)
Hemorrhage - (Hémorragie)
Hemorrhagic -
(Hémorragique)
Hemorrhagic stroke; cerebral
vascular accident -
(Hémorragie cérébrale)
Hemorrhoid - (Hémorroïde)
Hemostasis - (Hémostase)
Hemothorax - (Hémo thorax)
Heparin - (Héparine)
Hepatic - (Hépatique)
Hepatitis - (Hépatite)
Hepatobiliary - (Hépato

biliaire)
Hepatology - (Hépatologie)
Hepatomegaly; enlarged liver
- (Hépatomégalie)
Hepatosplenomegaly; enlarged
liver and spleen - (Hépato-
splénomégalie)
Hepatotoxicity - (Hépato
toxine)
Hereditary - (Héréditaire)
Hernia, having a - (Qui a une
hernie)
Hernia, hiatal - (Hernie
hiatale)
Hernia, inguinal - (Hernie
inguinale)
Hernia, strangulated - (Hernie
étranglée)
Hernia, umbilical - (Hernie
ombilicale)
Hernia; herniatiom - (Hernie)
Herniorrhaphy; hernia repair -
(Herniographie)
Herpangina - (Herpangine)
Herpes - (Herpès)
Herpes zoster - (Herpès
zoster, zona)
Herpetiforme dermatitis -
(Dermatite herpétiforme)
Heterogeneous -
(Hétérogène)
Heterosexual - (Hétérosexuel)
Heterosexuality -
(Hétérosexualité)
Hiatus - (Hiatus)

Hiccups - (Hoquet)
Hidden - (Caché (e))
Hide, to - (Cacher)
Hidradenitis - (Hydro adénite)
Hilum - (Hile)
Hip - (Hanche)
hip socket - (Acétabule)
Hirsutism - (Hirsutisme)
Histologist - (Histologique)
Histology - (Histologie)
Histoplasmosis -
(Histoplasmose)
HIV virus - (Virus de
l'immunodéficience Humaine,
VIH)
Hives - (Urticaire)
Hoarse - (Rauque, enroué (e))
Hoarseness - (Enrouement)
Hole - (Trou)
Home medical visit; housecall
- (Consultation médicale à
domicile)
Homeostasis - (Homéostasie)
Homicide - (Homicide)
Homologous - (Homologue)
Homosexual - (Homosexuel)
Homosexuality -
(Homosexualité)
Homozygote - (Homozygote)
Hookworm - (Ankylostome)
Horizontal - (Horizontal)
Hormonal - (Hormonal)
Hormone - (Hormone)
hormone - (hormone)
Hospital - (Hôpital)

Hospital - (Hôpital)
Hospital discharge - (Congé de l'hôpital)
Hospital stay - (Jours d'hospitalisation)
Hospital, children's - (Hôpital pédiatrique)
Hospital, city - (Hôpital municipal)
Hospital, general - (Hôpital général)
Hospital, military - (Hôpital militaire)
Hospital, rural - (Hôpital rural)
Hospitalization - (Hospitalisation)
Hospitalize - (Hospitaliser)
hosts - (hôtes)
Hot - (Chaud)
Hot water bottle - (Bouillotte)
Hour - (Heure)
House call - (Visite à domicile)
Human - (Humain)
Humerus - (Humérus)
Humoral; body fluids, pertaining to - (Humoral-relatifs aux humeurs du corps)
Hump - (Bosse)
Hunger - (Faim)
Hurt - (Fait mal)
hydatid cyst - (kyste hydatique)
Hydrate - (Hydrater)
Hydration - (Hydratation)
Hydrocephaly - (Hydrocéphalie)

Hydronephrosis - (Hydronéphrose)
Hydrophilic - (Hydrophile)
Hydrophobia - (Hydrophobie)
Hydropneumothorax - (Hydro-pneumothorax)
Hydropsy - (Hydropisie)
Hydrosalpinx - (Hydrosalpinx)
Hydrothorax - (Hydrothorax)
Hygiene - (Hygiène)
Hygienic - (Hygiénique)
Hymen - (Hymen)
Hyper - (Hyper)
Hyperacidity - (Hyper acidité)
Hyperactivity - (Hyperactivité)
Hyperbilirubinemia - (Hyperbilirrubinémie)
Hypercalcemia - (hypercalcémie)
Hypercholesterolemia - (Hypercholestérolémie)
Hyperemia - (Hyperémie)
Hyperesthesia - (Hyperesthésie)
Hyperfibrinemia - (Hyperfibrinémie)
Hyperglycemia - (Hyperglycémie)
Hyperhidrosis - (Hyperhydrose)
Hyperkalemia - (Hyperpotassémie)
Hyperkinesia - (Hypercinésie)
Hyperlipidemia - (Hyperlipidémie)
Hyperopia (farsightedness) -

(Hypermétropie)
Hyperopia (farsightedness) -
(Hypermétropie)
Hyperplasia - (Hyperplasie)
Hyperplasia - (Hyperplasie)
Hyperpnea - (Hyperpnée)
Hyperreactivity - (Hyper
réactivité)
Hyperreflexia -
(Surrréflectivité)
Hypersecretion - (Hyper
sécrétion)
Hypersensitivity -
(Hypersensibilité)
Hypertension (high blood
pressure) - (Hypertension)
Hypertensive - (Hypertendu)
Hypertensive - (Hypertenseur)
Hyperthermia -
(Hyperthermie)
Hyperthermia -
(Hyperthermie)
Hyperthyroidism -
(Hyperthyroïdie)
Hypertonia - (Hypertonie)
Hypertrophy - (Hypertrophie)
Hyperuricemia -
(Hyperuricémie)
Hyperventilation - (Hyper
ventilation)
Hypervolemia -
(Hypervolémie)
Hypoactive - (Hypo-activité)
Hypochondria -
(Hypochondrie)

Hypochondriac -
(Hypochondriaque)
Hypodermic - (Hypodermique)
Hypodermis - (Hypoderme)
Hypofunction (insufficiency) -
(Hypofonction)
Hypoglossal - (Hypoglosse)
Hypoglycemia -
(Hypoglycémie)
Hypoglycemic -
(Hypoglycémique)
Hypogonadism (low
testosterone) -
(Hypogonadisme)
Hypokalemia -
(Hypopotassémie)
Hypokinesia - (Hypocinésie)
Hyponatremia - (Hyposodé)
Hypoperfusion -
(Hypoperfusion)
Hypophysis, of the; pituitary,
of the - (Hypophysaire)
Hypophysis; pituitary gland -
(Hypophyse)
Hypopituitarism -
(Hypopituitarisme)
Hyporeflexia -
(Hyporéflectivité)
Hypotension (low blood
pressure) - (Hypotension)
Hypotensive - (Hypotendu (e))
Hypotensive - (hypotension)
Hypothalamus -
(Hypothalamus)
Hypothermia - (Hypothermie)

Hypothyroidism - (Hypotyroïdisme)
Hypotonia - (Hypotonie)
Hypoventilation (respiratory depression) - (Hypoventilation)
Hypovolemia - (Hypovolémie)
Hypoxia - (Hypoxie)
Hypoxic - (Hypoxique)
Hysterectomy - (hystérectomie)
Hysteria - (Hystérie)
Hysterical - (Hystérique)

~ I ~

Iatrogen - (Iatrogenie)
Iatrogenic - (Iatrogénique)
Iatrogenic - (Iatrogènique)
Ice - (Glace)
Ice bag - (Sac de glace)
Ichtyosis - (Ichthyose)
Idea, same - (Idée identique)
Identical twins - (Jumeaux identiques)
Identification - (Identification)
Idiopathic - (Idiopathique)
Idiosyncrasy - (Idiosyncrasie)
Ignorance; lack of knowledge - (Méconnaissance)
Ignore; unaware of, to be - (Ignorer)
Ileitis - (Iléite)
Ileum - (Iléon)
Ileum - (Iléon)

Iliac - (Iliaque)
ill, to be - (Souffrir)
Illiterate - (Analphabète)
Image - (Image)
Imbecile - (Imbécile)
Immature - (Immature)
Immobilization - (Immobilisation)
Immune - (Réfractaire a' certaines maladies)
Immunity - (Immunité)
immunity - (l'immunité)
Immunization - (immunisation)
Immunology - (Immunologie)
Immunosuppressant - (Immunosuppresseur)
Immunosuppression - (Immuno-dépression)
Impalpable - (Impalpable)
Impenetrable - (Impénétrable)
Imperfect - (Imparfait)
Impetigo - (Impétigo)
Implant, to - (Implanter)
Implication - (Implication)
Importance - (Importance)
Importance - (Importance)
Impotence - (Impuissance)
Impregnate, to - (Imprégner)
Impregnation - (imprégnation)
Improbable; unlikely - (Improbable)
Improvement - (Amélioration)
Impulse - (Impulsion, élan)
Impure - (Impur (e))
Impurity - (Impureté)

In addition - (En plus)
In bad shape - (En mauvais état)
In front of - (Devant)
In situ - (In situ, sur le terrain)
In vitro - (In vitro)
In vivo - (In vivo)
Inaccessible - (Inaccessible)
Inactive - (Inactif (ive))
Inadequate - (Inadéquat (e))
Inanition - (Inanition)
Inanition; fasting - (Privation d'aliment pendantlongtemps)
Incapable - (Incapable)
Incarceration - (Incarcération)
Incidence - (Incidence)
Incision - (Fissure)
Incisive - (Incisif (ive))
Inclined - (Incliné)
Include, to - (Inclure)
Included - (Inclus)
Incoherent - (Incohérent)
Incompatible - (Incompatible)
Incompetent - (Incompétent)
Incontinence - (Incontinence)
Incontinent - (Incontinent)
Incubation - (Incubation)
incubation - (incubation)
incubation - (incubation)
Incubator - (Couveuse)
Incurable - (Incurable)
Index finger - (Index)
Indicate, to; prescribe, to - (indiquer)

Indicated; specified - (Indiqué)
Indication; instruction; order - (Indication)
Indigestible - (Indigeste)
Indigestion - (Indigestion)
Indigestion - (Indigestion)
Indirect - (Indirect (e))
Indispensable - (Indispensable)
Individual - (Individuel)
Induction - (Induction)
Inebriated - (Ivre)
Inefficient - (Inefficace)
Inert - (Inerte)
Inertia - (Inertie)
Infancy - (Enfance)
Infant Mortality rate - (Taux de mortalité infantile)
Infant, premature - (Enfant prématuré)
Infantile development - (Développement de l'enfant)
Infarct - (Infarctus)
Infect, to - (Infecter)
Infected - (Infecté (e))
Infection - (Infection)
infection - (infection)
Infection, acute - (Infection aiguë)
Infection, chronic - (Infection chronique)
Infection, community acquired - (Infection acquise dans la communauté)

Infection, minimal contact - (Infection au contact minime)
Infection, opportunistic - (Infection opportuniste)
Infection, subclinical - (Infection sous clinique)
Infectious - (Infectieux (se))
Infectious agent - (Agent infectieux)
infectious disease - (maladie infectieuse)
Infectious disease; transmissible - (Maladie infectieuse,transmissible)
infertile - (infertiles)
Infertility - (Infertilité)
Infestation - (Infestation)
Infiltrated - (Infiltré (e))
Infiltration - (Infiltration)
Infirmary - (Infirmerie)
Inflamed - (Enflé (e))
inflamed gland - (Adénite)
Inflammation - (Inflammation)
inflammation - (inflammation)
Inflammation of fingers - (Dactylite, inflammation dudoigt)
Influenza - (Influenza)
Information - (Information)
Information; data - (Données)
Infraclavicular - (Infra claviculaire)
Infrared - (Infrarouge)
Infusion - (Infusion)
Ingest; consume - (ingérer)

Ingestion of medication - (Ingestion de médicament)
Inguinal - (Inguinal)
Ingurgitated - (Ingurgité(e))
Inhalation; breath - (Inhalation)
Inhale - (Inspiration)
Inhale, to - (Inhaler)
Inhaler - (Inhalateur)
Inheritance; heredity, to - (Héritage)
Inhibition - (Inhibition)
Initial dose - (Première dose, dose initiale)
Inject, to - (Injecter)
Injection - (Injection)
Injection, subcutaneous - (Injection sous-cutanée)
Injured person - (Accidenté(e))
Innate; inborn - (Inné)
Innervated - (Innervé (e))
Innervation - (Innervation)
Inoculation - (Inoculation)
Inoperable - (Inopérable)
Inorganic - (Inorganique)
Inotropic - (Inotropique)
Insane - (Fou)
Insect - (Insecte)
Insect control - (Contrôle d'insectes)
insecticide - (insecticide)
Insensitive - (Insensible)
Insert, to - (Insérer)
Insertion - (Insertion)
Inside - (A l'intérieur, en

dedans)
Inside - (Dedans)
Insolation - (Insolation)
Insoluble - (Insoluble)
Insomnia - (Insomniaque)
Insomniac - (Atteinte
d'insomnie)
Inspect, to - (Faire une
inspection)
Inspection - (Inspection)
Instillation - (Instillation)
Instrumental -
(Instrumentale)
Insufficiency - (Insuffisance)
Insulin - (Insuline)
Intelligence - (Intelligence)
Intensity - (Intensité)
Intention - (Intention)
Interaction - (Interaction)
Interaction of medications -
(Interaction des médicaments)
Intercostal - (Intercostal)
Intercurrent - (Intercurrent)
Interference - (Interférence)
Intermediary - (Intermédiaire)
Intermittent - (Intermittent)
Internal - (Interne)
Interrupt, to - (Interrompre)
Interstitial - (Interstitiel)
Interval - (Intervalle)
Intervention - (Intervention)
Intervention, surgical -
(Intervention chirurgicale)
Intervertebral -
(intervertébral)

Intestinal - (Intestinale)
Intestine - (Intestin)
intestine - (intestin)
Intestine, large - (Gros
intestin)
Intestine, small - (Intestin
grêle)
Intolerance - (Intolérance)
Intoxication; poisoning -
(Intoxication)
Intra abdominal - (Intra-
abdominal)
Intracranial - (Intracrânien)
Intramuscular -
(Intramusculaire)
Intraocular - (Intraoculaire)
Intrauterine - (Intra-utérin)
Intrauterine device; IUD -
(Stérilet)
Intravenous -
(Intraveineux(se))
Intravenous drugs - (Drogues
intraveineuses)
Intrinsic; inherent -
(Intrinsèque)
Introduce, to - (Introduire)
Introflection - (Introflexion)
Introitus - (Introduit)
Intromission - (Intromission)
Introspection - (Introspection)
Intubation - (Intubation)
Intubator - (Introducteur)
Invador - (Envahisseur)
Invagination - (Invagination)
Investigation; research -

(Recherche, investigation)
Invoice; bill - (Facture)
Involution - (Involution)
Iodine - (Iode)
Ionization - (Ionisation)
Iris - (Iris)
Iritis - (Iritis)
Iron - (Fer)
Irregular; erratic - (Irrégulier)
Irrigation - (Irrigation)
Irritant - (Irritant)
Irritate, to - (Irriter)
Irritation - (Irritation)
Ischemia - (Ischémie)
Ischemic - (Ischémique)
isolate - (isoler)
Isolate, to - (Isoler, éloigner)
Isotonic - (Isotonique)
Itch, to - (Piquer)
Itching - (Démangeaison.
picotement)
Itching, pruritus -
(Démangeaison,
picotement,prurit)

~ J ~

Jaundice - (Jaunisse)
Jaundice, neonatal - (Jaunisse
du nouveau-né)
Jaundice, newborn - (Jaunisse
du nouveau-né)
Jaundiced - (Ictérique, qui a la
jaunisse)
Jaw, lower - (Maxillaire

inférieur)
Jaw, upper - (Maxillaire
supérieur)
Jaw; jawbone - (Mâchoire)
Jaw; maxillary - (Maxillaire)
Jejunitis - (Inflammation du
jéjunum)
Jejunum - (Jéjunum)
Jelly - (Gelée)
Join - (Unir)
Joint - (Articulation)
Joint - (Articulation)
joint - (commune)
Jugal - (Malaire, jugal)
Jugular - (Jugulaire)
jugular - (La jugulaire)
Juice - (Jus)
Juice - (Jus)
Jump, to - (Sauter)
Juxtaposition - (Juxtaposition)

~ K ~

Kanamycin - (Kanamycine)
Karyotype - (Caryotype)
keep warm - (Abriter)
Keloid - (Chéloïde)
Keratin - (Kératine)
Keratinized - (Kératinisée)
Keratitis - (Kératite)
Keratoconjunctivitis - (Kérato-
conjonctivite)
Keratolytic - (Kératolytique)
Keratosis - (Kératose)
Ketoacidosis - (Cetoacidose)

Ketosis - (Cetose)
Kidney - (Rein)
Kidney pain - (Mal aux reins)
Kidney stone - (Calcul rénal)
Kilo; kilogram - (Kilo, kilogramme)
Kilocalorie - (Kilocalorie)
Kilometer - (Kilomètre)
Kind; nice (a person is...) - (Sympathique)
Kiss, to - (Embrasser)
Knee - (Genou)
Knot - (Nœud)
Know, to - (Savoir)
Know, to; meet, to - (Connaître, savoir)
Knowledge - (Connaissance)
Knuckle - (Jointure des doigts)
Kwashiorkor - (Kwashiorkor)
Kyphosis - (Cyphose)

~ L ~

Lab technician - (Technicien de laboratoire, laborantin)
Labial - (Labial)
Laboratory - (Laboratoire)
Laboratory Technician - (Technicien de laboratoire)
Labyrinthitis - (Labyrinthite)
Laceration - (Lacération)
Lack of coordination - (Incoordination)
Lack of; deficiency - (Carence)

Lack; deficiency - (Manque)
Lacrimal sac - (Poche lacrymale)
Lactate, to - (Allaiter, téter)
Lactation - (Allaitement)
Lactose - (Lactose)
Lame - (Boiteux)
lame - (boiteux)
laminitis - (fourbure)
Lancet - (Lancette)
Language - (Langue)
Language; speech - (Langage)
Laparoscopy - (Laparoscopie)
Laparotomy - (Laparotomie)
Lard - (Saindoux)
Large - (Grand)
Larva - (Larve)
larva - (larve)
Larvae - (Larves)
Laryngitis - (Laryngite)
Laryngography - (Radiographie du larynx)
Laryngorrhagia; hemorrhage from the larynx - (Hémorragie du larynx)
Laryngoscope - (Laryngoscope)
Laryngoscopy - (Laryngoscopie)
Laryngospasm - (Spasme du larynx)
Larynx - (Larynx)
Last - (Dernier (ère))
Last name - (Nom de famille)
Latency - (Latence)

Lateral - (Latéral)
Latrine - (Latrines)
latrine - (latrines)
Laugh - (Rire)
Lavage - (Lavement)
Lax - (Détendu (e))
Laxative - (Laxatif (ive))
Laxative - (Purgatif (ve))
laxative - (laxatif)
Laxity, laxness - (Laxisme)
Lay down, to - (Coucher)
Lead (noun) - (Plomb)
Leaf; sheet of paper - (Feuille)
Leave, to - (Sortir)
Left - (Gauche)
Left hand - (Main gauche)
Leg - (Jambe)
legume - (plantes légumineuses)
Length - (Longueur)
Lengthen, to; longer, to get - (S'allonger, rallonger, prolonger)
Lens - (Cristallin)
Lens; eyeglasses - (Lente, Lentilles)
Leper - (Lépreux)
Leprosy - (Lèpre)
Lesion; injury - (Lésion, blessure)
Lethal - (Mortel)
Lethargy - (Léthargie)
Leukemia - (Leucémie)
Leukocyte - (Leucocyte)
Leukocytosis - (Leucocytose)
Leukopenia - (Leucopénie)

Leukoplasia - (Leucoplasie)
Leukorrhea - (Leucorrhée – pertes blanches)
Level; standard - (Niveau)
Libido - (Libido)
Library - (Bibliothèque)
Lichenification - (Lichénification)
Lidocaine - (Lidocaïne)
Lie down, to; go to bed, to - (Se coucher)
Life - (Vie)
Life expectancy - (Espérance de vie)
Lifestyle - (Style de vie)
Ligament - (Ligament)
Ligation - (Ligature)
Ligation, tubal - (Ligature des trompes)
Light - (Lumière)
Light; mild; low-grade - (Léger(ère))
Light; slight; gentle - (Léger)
Limb - (Extrémité)
Limb asleep e.g.: My leg is asleep - (Membre endormi)
Limb; member - (Membre)
Limp - (Boiter, clocher)
Linear - (Linéal)
Lining; covering - (Revêtement)
Lip; labium - (Lèvre)
Lipid - (Lipide)
Lipoma - (Lipome)
Liposoluble - (Liposoluble)
Liquid - (Liquide)

Liquor - (Liqueur)
Liter - (Litre)
Lithiasis - (Lithiase)
Lithic; stones, pertaining to -
(Lithique)
Little - (Peu)
Little finger; pinky -
(Auriculaire)
Liver - (Foie)
Lobule; lobe - (Lobule)
Local - (Local)
local anaesthetic -
(anesthésique local)
Localization - (Localisation)
Localized - (Localisé)
Lochia - (Lochies)
Locomotion - (Locomotion)
Lodge a foreign body, to -
(Loger un corps étranger)
Long - (Long)
Longevity - (Longévité)
Long-lived - (Très âgé)
Long-term care - (Soin à long
terme)
Look for, to - (Chercher)
Lordosis - (Lordose)
Lose blood, to - (Perdre du
sang)
Lose weight; become thin -
(Maigrir)
Lose, to - (Perdre)
Loss of consciousness - (Perte
de la connaissance)
Loss of voice - (Perte de la
voix)

Lotion - (Lotion)
Low - (Bas(se))
Low grade fever -
(Légèrement fiévreux)
Lower limb - (Extrémité
inférieure)
Lower, to - (Descendre)
Lubricant - (Lubrifiant)
Lumbago - (Lumbago)
Lumbar - (Lombaire)
Lump - (Bosse)
Lunch - (Déjeuner, dîner,
lunch)
Lung - (Poumon)
Lung cavity - (Caverne
pulmonaire)
Lupus - (Lupus)
Lying - (Décubitus)
lymph - (Supprimer la lymphe
)
lymph node - (ganglionnaire)
lymph vessel - (vaisseau
lymphatique)
Lymphadenitis -
(Lymphangite)
Lymphadenopathy -
(Lymphadénopathie)
Lymphangitis - (Lymphangite)
Lymphatic ganglion -
(Ganglion lymphatique)
Lymphocyte - (Lymphocyte)
Lymphocytopenia -
(Lymphocytopénie)
Lymphocytosis -
(Lymphocytose)

Lymphoma - (Lymphome)
Lysis - (Quand un cellule meure acause la membrane est brisée)

~ M ~

Macerated - (Pultacé(e))
Maceration - (Macération)
Macrocephaly - (Macrocéphalie)
Macrocyte - (Macrocyte)
Macroglossia - (Macroglossie)
Macrolide - (Macrolide)
Macrophage - (Macrophage)
Macular degeneration - (Dégénérescence maculaire)
Macule - (Tache)
Maculopapular - (Maculopapulaire)
Maintenance dose - (Dose de maintenance, demaintien)
Malabsorption - (Mauvaise absorption)
Malabsorption, intestinal - (Mauvaise absorption intestinale)
Malaise - (Malaise, douleur)
Malar; cheek, relating to the - (Malaire)
Malaria - (Malaria)
Malaria - (Paludisme)
Male - (Genre masculin)
Male; man - (Garçon)
Malformation - (Malformation)

Malignant - (Maligne)
Malleolus - (Cheville)
Malnourished - (Malnutri (e), sous-alimenté(e))
Malnourished - (Sous-alimenté (e))
Malnutrition - (Malnutrition)
Malnutrition - (Malnutrition)
Mammary - (Mammaire)
Mammogram; mammography - (Mammographie)
Man - (Homme)
Management, illness - (Gestion ou contrôle de la maladie)
Mandible; jaw - (Mâchoire)
Maneuver - (Manœuvre)
mange - (mange maladie)
Mania - (Manie)
Manic-depressive - (Maniaco-dépressif (ive))
Manifestation - (Manifestation)
Manometer - (Éprouvette)
Marasmus; wasting - (Marasme)
March; progress - (Marche)
Marijuana - (Marihuana)
Mark; brand - (Marque)
Married - (Marié(e))
Marrow - (Moelle)
Masculine - (Masculin)
Mask - (Masque)
Mass - (Masse)
Massage - (Massage)
Massage therapist; masseur/masseuse -

(Masseur)
Masseter - (Masséter)
Mastectomy - (Mastectomie)
Mastitis - (Mastite)
mastitis - (mastite)
Mastocyte - (Mastocyte)
Mastodynia; mastalgia -
(Mastodynie, mastalgie)
Mastoid - (Mastoïde)
Mastoiditis - (Mastoïdite)
Maternal care - (Soin
maternel)
Maternity - (Maternité)
Matron - (Matrone, femme-
sage)
Mattress - (Matelas)
Maturation - (Maturation)
Maximum - (Maximal (e))
Measles - (Rougeole)
Measure - (Mesurer)
Meat - (Viande)
Meatus - (Méat)
Mechanism - (Mécanisme)
Meconium - (Méconium)
Mediastinum - (Médiastin)
Medical advance - (Progrès
médical)
Medical assistance -
(Assistance médicale)
Medical care - (Soins
médicaux)
Medical certificate - (Certificat
médical)
Medical check-up - (Bilan de
santé, check-up)

Medical Diploma - (Diplôme
de médecine)
Medical ethic - (Éthique
médicale)
Medical examination -
(Auscultation médicale)
Medical File - (Dossier
médical)
Medical school - (École de
médecine)
Medical school - (Faculté de
médecine)
Medical specialist - (Spécialité
médicale)
Medical student - (Étudiant en
médecine)
Medical technology -
(Technologie médicale)
Medication - (Médication)
Medication abuse - (Abus de
médicaments)
Medication, psychiatric -
(Psychotrope)
Medication, to give a -
(Administrer un médicament)
Medicinal - (Médicinal)
Medicinal product - (Produit
médicinal)
Medicine - (Médecine)
Medicine - (Médicament)
Medicine cabinet; medicine kit
- (Trousse à pharmacie,
armoire)
Medicine dependence -
(Dépendance du médicament)

Medicine, community - (Médecine communautaire)
Medicine, family - (Médecine familiale)
Medicine, preventative - (Médecine préventive)
Medicine, sport - (Médecine sportive)
Medicine, traditional - (Médecine traditionnelle)
Medicine; remedy(home remedy) - (Médicament)
Medium; half - (Milieu, demi)
Medullary - (Médullaire)
Megacolon - (Mégacôlon)
Megakaryocyte - (Mégacaryocyte)
Meiosis - (Méiose)
Melanoma - (Mélanome)
melanoma - (mélanome)
Melena - (Méléna)
Membrane - (Membrane)
Membrane, cellular - (Membrane cellulaire)
Memory - (Mémoire)
Menarche - (Menarchie)
Meninges - (Méninges)
Meningitis - (Méningite)
Meningoencephalitis - (Méningo-encéphalite)
Menopause - (Ménopause)
Menopause - (Ménopause)
Menorraghia - (Hyperménorrhée)
Menorrhagia - (Ménorragie)
Menstrual - (Menstruel)

Menstrual cycle - (Cicle menstrual)
Menstrual period; rule; ruler - (Règle)
Menstruation - (Règles, menstruation)
Mental - (Mental)
Mental disorders - (Troubles mentaux)
Mesentery - (Mésentère)
Mesogastrium - (Mésogastre)
Metabolism - (Métabolisme)
Metabolite - (Métabolite)
Metacarpus - (Métacarpe)
Metaphysis - (Métaphyse)
Metaplasia - (Métaplasie)
Metastasis - (Métastase)
Metastatic - (Métastatique)
Metastisized cancer - (Cancer disséminé)
Metatarsal - (Éminence métatarsienne)
Metrorrhagia - (Métrorragie)
Microbe - (Microbe)
microbe - (microbe)
Microbiology - (Microbiologie)
Microorganism - (Microorganisme)
Microscope - (Microscope)
microscope - (microscope)
Microscopic - (Microscopique)
Midnight - (Minuit)
Midwife - (Sage femme, matrone)
Migraine - (Migraine)
Migraine - (Migraine)

Milk - (Lait)
Milk, pertaining to; dairy product - (Laitier)
Milligram - (Milligramme)
mineral   - (minérale)
Mineralocorticoid - (Minéralocorticoïde)
Minimal - (Minimal)
Minor; smaller or less than - (Plus petit que, mineur)
Minute - (Minute)
mite - (Acarus)
mite - (mite)
Mitosis - (Mitose)
Mitral - (Mitral)
Mitral valve stenosis - (Sténose mitral)
Mixture - (Mélange)
Mobility - (Mobilité)
Mobilization - (Mobilisation)
Moderate - (Modéré (e))
Modification - (Modification)
modify - (Altérer)
modify - (changer)
modify - (modifier)
modify - (troubler)
Molar - (Molaire)
Molars - (Molaires)
Mole - (Môle)
Molecule - (Molécule)
Moment - (Moment)
Moment - (Moment)
Monitor - (Moniteur)
Monitor, to; to follow - (Suivre)

Monitoring - (Monitorage)
Monitoring (following) - (Suivi)
Monoarticular - (Mono-articulaire)
Monocyte - (Monocyte)
Mononucleosis, infectious - (Mononucléose infectieuse)
Monoplegia - (Monoplégie)
Monotherapy - (Mono-thérapie)
Mood - (État d'esprit)
Morbidity - (Morbidité)
More - (Plus)
More than - (Plus grand que, majeur)
Moribund - (Moribond (e))
Morphine - (Morphine)
Mortal - (Mortel)
Mortality - (Mortalité)
Mortality rate - (Taux de mortalité)
Mortality, infant - (Mortalité infantile)
Mortality, maternal - (Mortalité maternelle)
Mosquito - (Moustique)
Mosquito control - (Contrôle de moustiques)
Mother - (Maman)
Mother - (Mère)
Mother, single - (Mère célibataire)
Motility - (Motilité)
Motility, intestinal - (Motilité intestinale)

Motivation - (Motivation)
Motor - (Moteur)
Mouth - (Bouche)
Mouthpiece; snack (reg) - (Bec)
Move, to - (Bouger)
Movement - (Mouvement)
Mucocutaneous - (Mucocutané)
Mucolytic - (Mucolytique)
Mucous - (Muqueuse)
mucous membrane - (muqueuse)
mucus - (mucus)
Mucus; snot - (Morve, crotte de nez)
Multifactorial - (Multi-factoriel)
Multifocal - (Multi-focal)
Multipara - (Multipare)
Multiple - (Multiple)
Multiple pregnancy - (Grossesse multiple, gémellaire)
Mumps - (Oreillon)
Murmur - (Murmure)
Murmur - (Souffle)
Murmur respiratory; vesicular breath sounds - (Murmure respiratoire, murmure vésiculaire)
Murmur, heart - (Souffle cardiaque)
Murmur, heart; cardiac murmur - (Murmure cardiaque)
Murmur, systolic - (Murmure systolique)

Muscle - (Muscle)
muscle - (musculaires)
Muscle, smooth - (Muscle lisse)
Muscular - (Musculaire)
Muscular contraction - (Contraction musculaire)
Musculature - (Musculature)
Musculoskeletal - (Muscle-squelettique)
Mutation - (Mutation)
Mute - (Muet)
Mutism - (Mutisme)
Myalgia - (Myalgie)
Myasthenia - (Myasthénie)
Mycobacteria - (Micro-bactérie)
mycoplasmav Microbes similar to bacteria . - (mycoplasmav microbes semblables à des bactéries (p. 88).)
Mycosis - (Mycosis)
Mycotic - (Mycotique)
Mydriasis - (Mydriase)
Mydriatic - (Mydriatique)
Myelin - (Myéline)
Myelitis - (Myélite)
Myelography - (Myélographie)
Myeloma - (Myélome)
Myelomeningocele (MMC) - (Myeloméningocèles)
myiasis - (myiasis)
Myocarditis - (Myocardite)
Myocardium - (Myocarde)
Myology - (Myologie)
Myoma - (Myome)

Myopathia - (Myopathie)
Myopia - (Myopie)
Myosis - (Myosis)
Myotic - (Myotique)
Myxedema - (Myxœdème)
Myxomatosis - (Myxomatose)

~ N ~

Nail - (Ongle)
Name - (Nom)
Nap - (Sieste)
Narcotic - (Narcotique)
Nasopharyngitis - (Rinopharyngite)
Nasopharynx - (Rhinopharynx)
Nasopharynx - (Rinopharynx)
Natural catasrophe - (Catastrophe naturelle)
Nauseous - (Nausées)
navel - (nombril)
Near; Fence; Hedge - (Près)
Nearby - (Proche)
Nebulization - (Nébulisation)
Nebulizer - (Nébuliseur)
Neck - (Cou)
Neck, nape of the - (Nuque)
Necrosis - (Nécrose)
Needle - (Aiguille)
Negative - (Négatif (ive))
Negatoscope - (Négatoscope)
Negligence, medical - (Négligence médicale)
Neighbor - (Voisin (e))

Nemathelminthe - (Némathelminthe)
Nematode - (Nématode)
nematodes - (nématodes)
Neonatal - (Néonatal)
Neoplastic - (Néoplasique)
Nephrectomy - (Néphrectomie)
Nephritic - (Néphrétique)
Nephritis - (Néphrite)
Nephrolithiasis - (Lithiase rénale)
Nephrology - (Néphrologie)
Nephropathy - (Néphropathie)
Nephrosis - (Néphrose)
Nephrotoxic - (Néphrotoxique)
Nerve - (Nerf)
Nerve, trigeminal - (Trigémellaire)
nerves - (nerfs)
Nervous - (Nerveux)
Nervous breakdown - (Crise nerveuse)
Nervous Breakdown - (Crise nerveuse)
Nervous breakdown - (Dépression nerveuse)
Nervous exhaustion - (Neurasthénie)
Nervousness - (Nervosité)
Net; network - (Réseau)
Neural - (Neural)
Neuralgia - (Névralgie)
Neuritis - (Névrite)
Neurobiology -

(Neurobiologie)
Neuroleptic - (Neuroleptique)
Neurologist - (Neurologue)
Neurology - (Neurologie)
Neuromuscular -
(Neuromusculaire)
Neuron - (Neurone)
Neuronal - (Relatif aux
neurones)
Neuropathology -
(Neuropathologie)
Neuropathy - (Neuropathie)
Neuropsychiatry -
(Neuropsychiatrie)
Neurosis - (Névrose)
Neurosurgeon -
(Neurochirurgien)
Neurosurgery -
(Neurochirurgie)
Neurotic - (Névrotique)
Neurotoxic - (Neurotoxique)
Neurotropism -
(Neurotropisme)
Neutralization -
(Neutralisation)
Neutropenia - (Neutropénie)
Neutrophilia - (Neutrophilie)
Never - (Jamais)
Newborn - (Nouveau-né)
Newborn - (Nouveau-né (e))
Next - (Suivant)
Next to - (Prochain (e))
Niacine - (Niacinamide)
Nicotine - (Nicotine)
Nicotinic - (Nicotinique)
Nicturia - (Nycturie)

Night - (Nuit)
Ninth - (Neuvième)
Nipple - (Mamelon)
Nipple - (Mamelon)
Nitroglycerine -
(Nitroglycérine)
Nodular - (Nodulaire)
Nodule - (Nodule)
Noise - (Bruit)
Non-compliance; non-
fulfillment - (Non- respect)
Non-steroidal anti-
inflammatories; NSAIDs -
(Anti-inflammatoire non
stéroïdien)
Noon - (Midi)
Noradrenaline -
(Noradrénaline)
Normal - (Normal)
Normal intestinal flora - (Flore
intestinale normale)
Normalization -
(Normalisation)
Normoglycemia - (Qui a une
glycémie normale)
Normotensive - (Qui a une
tension normale)
Normothermia - (Qui a une
température nor-male)
Nose - (Nez)
Nosography - (Nosographie)
Nosology - (Nosologie)
Nostalgia - (Nostalgie)
Nostril - (Fosse nasale)
Notalgia - (Notalgie)
Note, to - (Noter)

Nothing - (Rien)
Notification - (Notification)
Nourish, to; feed, to -
(Nourrir)
Novocaine - (Novocaïne)
Now - (Maintenant)
NPO; fasting - (Prohibition
d'aliments)
Nucleic acid - (Acide
nucléique)
Nucleus - (Noyau)
Null - (Nul(le))
Nullipara - (Nullipare)
Numbed; sedated -
(Engourdi(e), endormi(e))
Number - (Numéro)
Nurse - (Infirmier(ière))
Nurse, wet - (Nourrice)
Nurse's Assistant - (Auxiliaire,
aide infirmière)
Nursing home - (Foyer pour
personnes âgées)
Nursing infant - (Nourrisson)
Nutrient - (Nutriment)
Nutrition - (Nutrition)
Nutritional analysis - (Analyse
des aliments)
Nutritional deficiency -
(Déficience nutritionnelle)
Nutritious - (Nutritif (ive))
nymph - (nymphe)
Nymphomania -
(Nymphomanie)
Nystagmus - (Nystagmus)
Nystatin - (Nistatine)

~ O ~

Obese - (Obèse)
Obesity - (Obésité)
Objective - (Objectif)
Obliteration - (Oblitération)
Observation - (Observation)
Observation; vigilance -
(Vigilance)
Observe, to - (Observer)
Obsession - (Obsession)
Obsolete - (Obsolète)
Obstetric services;
gynecological services -
(Service de gynécologie
etobstétrique)
Obstetrician - (Obstétricien)
Obstetrics - (Obstétrique)
Obstruction - (Obstruction)
Obtuse - (Obtus)
Occasional - (Occasionnel)
Occipital - (Occipital)
Occlude - (Occlure)
Occlusion, to cause -
(Occlusion)
Ocular - (Oculaire)
Odontoblastoma -
(Odontoblastome)
Odontocele - (Odontocèles)
Odontologist - (Odontologiste)
Odontology - (Odontologie)
Odontoma - (Odontome)
Odontophobia -
(Odontophobie)

Odor - (Odeur)
Odorless - (Inodore)
Odyphagia - (Odinophagie)
oesophagus - (oesophage)
oestrus - (oestrus)
official document - (Acte)
Ointment - (Onguent)
Ointment - (Pommade)
Old age - (Vieillesse)
Old man; old woman -
(Vieux/vieille, personne âgée)
Oligomenorrhea -
(Oligomenorrhée)
Oliguria - (Oligurie)
omasum - (omasum)
Omphalitis - (Omphalite)
Oncology - (Oncologie,
cancérologie)
Oncotic - (Oncotique)
One-eyed - (Borgne)
One-handed - (Manchot)
One-sided; unilateral -
(Unilatéral (e))
Opacity - (Opacité)
Open - (Ouvert)
Open, to - (Ouvrir)
Opening - (Ouverture)
Operable - (Opérable)
Operate, to - (Opérer)
Operating room - (Salle
d'opération)
Operation - (Opération)
Operation, risky - (Opération
risquée)
Ophthalmia - (Ophtalmie)
Ophthalmic - (Ophtalmique)

Ophthalmologic -
(Ophtalmologique)
Ophthalmologist -
(Ophtalmologue)
Ophthalmologist -
(Ophtalmologue)
Ophthalmology -
(Opthalmologie)
Ophthalmoscope -
(Ophtalmoscope)
Ophthalmoscopy -
(Ophtalmoscopie)
Opiate - (Opiacé)
Opinion, to give an - (Opiner)
Opisthotonos - (Opisthotonos)
Opportunist - (Opportuniste)
Opportunity - (Opportunité)
Oppress - (Oppressif (ive))
Oppression - (Oppression)
Optical - (Optique)
Optimum - (Optimal)
Optometrist - (Optométriste)
Oral - (Oral)
Oral cavity - (Cavité orale)
Oral exam - (Examen oral)
Oral hygiene - (Hygiène
buccale)
Oral Rehydration Therapy
(ORT) - (Thérapie de
réhydratationorale)
Orally - (Voie orale)
Orbit - (Orbite)
Orbital - (Orbitaire, orbital)
Orchitis - (Orchite)
Organ - (Organe)
Organism - (Organisme)

organism - (organisme)
Organomegaly -
(Viscéromégalie)
Orgasm - (Orgasme)
Orientation - (Orientation)
Orifice - (Orifice)
Origin - (Origine)
Oropharynx - (Oropharynx)
Orthodontics - (Orthodontie)
Orthopedic - (Orthopédique)
Orthopnea - (Orthopnée)
Orthostatic - (Orthostatique)
Osmotic - (Osmotique)
Ossification - (Ossification)
Ostealgia - (Ostéalgie)
Osteitis - (Ostéite)
Ostemalacia - (Ostéomalacie)
Osteoarthritis - (Ostéo-
arthrite)
Osteoarthrosis - (Ostéo-
arthrose)
Osteocondritis -
(Ostéochondrose)
Osteodystrophy - (Ostéo-
dystrophie)
Osteolysis - (Ostéolyse)
Osteomyelitis - (Ostéomyélite)
Osteopathy - (Ostéopathie)
Osteophyte - (Ostéophyte)
Osteoplasty - (Ostéoplastie)
Osteoporosis - (Ostéoporose)
Osteosarcoma -
(Ostéosarcome)
Other - (Autre)
Otitis - (Otite)

Otology - (Otologie)
Otomycosis - (Oto-mycose)
Otorrhagia - (Otorragie)
Otorrhea - (Otorrhée)
Otosclerosis - (Otosclérose)
Otoscope - (Otoscope)
Ototoxic - (Oto-toxique)
Outside - (Dehors)
Outside of; out - (Dehors,
hors)
Ovary - (Ovaire)
ovary - (ovaire)
Overcrowded housing;
stacking; heaping;
accumulation - (Entassement)
Overdose - (Surdose)
Overweight - (Surpoids)
Overwhelmed - (Accablement)
Ovulate - (Ovuler)
Ovule; ovum; egg - (Ovule)
Own (as in his own, her own)
or to be correct; appropriate -
(Propre)
Oxigenotherapy -
(Oxygénothérapie)
Oxygen - (Oxygène)
oxygen - (l'oxygène)
Oxygen mask - (Masque
d'oxygène)
Oxygenated water - (Eau
oxygénée)
Oxygenation - (Oxygénation)
Oxymetry - (Oxymétrie)
Oxytocin - (Oxytocine)
oxytocin - (ocytocine)

~ P ~

Pacemaker - (Pacemaker, stimulateur cardiaque)
Pain - (Douleur)
Pain - (Douleur)
Painless - (Indolore)
Palate - (Palais)
Pale - (Pâle)
Pale, to become - (Pâlir)
Pale; livid - (Livide)
Palliate - (Apaiser, pallier)
Palliative - (Palliatif (ive))
Pallor - (Lividité)
Pallor - (Pâleur)
Palm - (Paume)
Palm of the hand - (Paume de la main)
Palpable - (Palpable)
Palpation - (Palpation)
Palpebral - (Palpébral)
Palpitation - (Palpitation)
Panacea - (Panacée)
Pan-American Health Organization - (Office Panaméricain de la Santé)
Pancreas - (Pancréas)
Pancreatitis - (Pancréatite)
Pancytopenia - (Pancytopénie)
Panniculitis - (Panniculite)
Panting; gasping - (Halètement)
Pap (soft food) - (Bouillie)
Paper; role - (Papier)
Papilledema - (Papillœdème)

Papule - (Papule, nodule)
Paracentesis - (Paracentèse)
Parainfluenza - (Para-influenza)
Parallel - (Parallèle)
Paralysis - (Paralyse)
paralysis - (Une paralysie)
Paralytic - (Paralytique)
Paralyze - (Paralyser)
Paralyzed - (paralytique)
Paramedic; paramedical - (Paramédical)
Parameter - (Paramètres)
Paranoia - (Paranoïa)
Paraphimosis - (Paraphimosis)
Paraplegia - (Paraplégie)
Paraplegic - (Paraplégique)
Parasite - (Acarus)
Parasite - (sarcopte de la gale)
parasite - (parasite)
Parasites - (Parasites)
Parasitic - (Parasitaire)
parasitic gastro-enteritis - (parasitaire gastro-entérite)
Parasitic worm - (Helminthe)
Parasitic worm infections - (Helminthiase)
Parasitism - (Parasitisme)
Parasitized - (Parasité (e))
Parasternal - (Parasternal)
Parasympathetic - (Parasympathique)
Parathyroid - (Parathyroïdes)
Parenchyma - (Parenchyme)
Parenteral - (Parentéral)

Paresis - (Parésie)
Paretic - (Parétique)
Parkinsonism -
(Parkinsonismes, variations
dumal de Parkinson)
Paronychia - (Paronichie)
Parotid - (Parotide)
Parotiditis (mumps) -
(Parotidite, oreillon)
Paroxysmal - (Paroxysmale)
Partial denture - (Dentition
partielle)
Particle - (Particule)
Partner - (Camarade,
collègue)
Partner - (Partenaire)
Parturient; woman in labor -
(Femmes en couches)
Passage - (Passage, billet)
Past - (Passé)
Paste (noun) - (Pâte)
Patella; kneecap - (Rotule)
Pathogen - (Pathogénie)
Pathogenic - (Pathogène)
Pathognomonic -
(Pathognomonique)
Pathologic - (Pathologique)
Pathophysiology -
(Physiopathologie)
Patient - (Patient)
Patient isolation - (Isolement
des patients)
Patient room - (Chambre de
malade)
Pause - (Pause)

Pectoral - (Pectoral)
Pediatric - (Pédiatrique)
Pediatrician - (Pédiatre)
Pediatrics - (Pédiatrie)
Pediculosis - (Pédiculose)
Pellagra - (Pellagre)
Pelvic - (Pelvien)
Pelvis - (Bassin, pelvis)
Penicillin - (Pénicilline)
Penis - (Pénis)
Penis - (Pénis, priape)
penis   - (pénis)
Peptic - (Peptique)
Perception - (Perception)
Percuss, to; to strike -
(Percuter)
Percussion - (Percussion)
Percutaneous - (Percutané
(e))
Perforation - (Perforation)
Perfusion - (Perfusion)
Perianal - (Péri-anal)
Periarthritis - (Périarthrite)
Pericarditis - (Péricardite)
Pericardium - (Péricarde)
Perinatal - (Périnatal)
Perineal - (Périnéal)
Perineum - (Périnée)
Period; menstruation -
(Période)
Periodic; newspaper or
magazine - (Périodique)
Peristalltic - (Péristaltique)
Peritoneal - (Péritonéal)
Peritoneum - (Péritoine)

Peritonitis - (Péritonite)
Peritonsillar abscess - (Abcès périamygdalien)
Permanent teeth - (Dents permanentes)
Permeable; not water proof - (Perméable)
Permission - (Permis)
Pernicious - (Pernicieux)
Persistent - (Persistant)
Personality - (Personnalité)
Perspire; sweat - (Transpirer)
Pertussis; whooping cough - (Coqueluche)
Pertussis; whooping cough - (Coqueluche)
Perversion - (Perversion)
Petechia - (Pétéchie)
Phagocyte - (Phagocyte)
Phagocytic - (Phagocytaire)
Phagocytize - (Phagocyter)
Phagocytosis - (Phagocytose)
Phalange - (Phalange)
Phallus - (Phallus)
Phamacist; druggist - (Pharmacien)
Pharmaceutical - (Pharmaceutique)
Pharmacodynamic - (Pharmacodynamique)
Pharmacodynamics - (Pharmacodynamie)
Pharmacokinetic - (Pharmacocinétique)
Pharmacologist - (Pharmacologue)

Pharmacology - (Pharmacologie)
Pharmacopoeia - (Pharmacopée)
Pharmacy; drug store - (Pharmacie)
Pharyngeal - (Pharyngé (e))
Pharyngitis - (Pharyngite)
Pharyngolaryngitis - (Pharyngo-laryngite)
Pharyngoscope - (Pharyngoscope)
Pharyngoscopy - (Pharyngoscopie)
Pharyngotomy - (Pharyngotomie)
Pharyngotonsillitis - (Pharyngo-amydalite)
Pharynx - (Pharynx)
Phase - (Phase)
Phenobarbitol - (Phénobarbital)
Phenomenon - (Phénomène)
Phenotype - (Phénotype)
Phenytoin - (Fénitöine)
Pheochromocytoma - (Phéochromocytome)
Phimosis - (Phimosis)
Phlebitis - (Phlébite)
Phleborrhagia - (Phléborragie)
Phlebothrombosis - (Phlébothrombose)
Phlebotomy - (Phlébotomie)
Phlegm; mucus - (Flegme)
Phlegmon, dental abcess - (Phlegmon, abcès dentaire)

Phobia - (Phobie)
Phocomelia - (Phocomélie)
Phosphate - (Phosphate)
Phosphaturia - (Phosphaturie)
Phosphorism - (Phosphorisme)
Photophobia - (Photophobie)
Photophobia - (Photophobie)
Photosensitive -
(Photosensible)
Photosensitivity -
(Photosensibilité)
Phototherapy -
(Photothérapie)
Phrenic - (Phrénique)
Physical exam - (Examen
physique)
Physical exercise - (Exercice
physique)
Physical therapist -
(Physiothérapeute)
Physical therapy -
(Physiothérapie)
Physical; physique -
(Physique)
Physiologic; physiological -
(Physiologique)
Physiology - (Physiologie)
Pierce, to; to puncture; to prick
- (Piquer)
Pigmentation - (Pigmentation)
Pill - (Comprimé)
Pill - (Pastille)
Pill (specifically a contraceptive
pill) - (Pilule)
Piloerection - (Piloérection)

Pimple; spot - (Bouton)
Pink - (Rose)
Pinkie; little finger -
(Auriculaire, petit doigt)
Pins and needles, sensation of;
ant hill - (Fourmillement)
Pityriasis - (Pityriasis)
Place - (Lieu, endroit)
Placebo - (Placebo)
Placenta - (Placenta)
placenta - (placenta)
Placenta abruptia - (Abruption
du placenta)
Plan; flat - (Plan, plat)
Planning, family; contraception
- (Planification familiale)
Planning, health -
(Planification de la santé)
Plant - (Plante)
Plasma - (Plasma)
Plaster - (Plâtre)
Plaster, to put in; cast, to -
(Mettre du plâtre)
Platelet - (Plaquette)
Plenitude; abundance -
(Plénitude)
plentiful - (Abondant)
Pleura - (Plèvre)
Pleural effusion -
(Épanchement pleural)
Pleuritis - (Pleurite)
Plexus - (Plexus)
pliers - (pinces)
Pneumococcus -
(Pneumocoque)

Pneumocystis jiroveci - (Pneumocystose)
Pneumonia - (Pneumonie)
Pneumonia - (Pneumonie)
pneumonia - (pneumonie)
Pneumopathy - (Pneumopathie)
Pneumorrhagia - (Pneumorragie)
Pneumothorax - (Pneumothorax)
Pocket dictionary - (Dictionnaire de poche)
Point; stitch; suture - (Point)
Point; tip - (Pointe)
Poison - (Poison)
Poison, to - (Empoisonner)
Poisoned - (Intoxiqué (e))
Poisoning - (Empoisonnement)
Poisoning, lead - (Saturnisme)
Poisonous - (Vénéneux(seuse), venimeux(euse))
Poliomyelitis - (Poliomyélite)
Pollen - (Pollen)
Polyarthritis - (Polyarthrite)
Polyclinic - (Polyclinique)
Polycythemia - (Polycythémie)
Polydipsia - (Polydipsie)
Polygamy - (Polygamie)
Polyhydramnios - (Polyhydramnios)
Polymorphic - (Polymorphique)
Polyp - (Polype)

Polyphagia - (Polyphagie)
Polysaccharide - (Polysaccharide)
Polyuria - (Polyurie)
Poor - (Pauvre)
Popliteal - (Poplité)
Population - (Population)
Position - (Position)
Positive - (Positif (ive))
Possible - (Possible)
Post-doctorate; graduate school (varies) - (Diplôme après licence)
Posterior - (Postérieur)
Posterior fontanel - (Fontanelle postérieure)
Postmenopausal - (Post-ménopausique)
Postoperative - (Postopératoire)
Post-operative care - (Soin post-opératoire)
Postpartum period - (Suite de couches)
Postprandial - (Postprandial)
Posture - (Posture)
Potable - (Potable)
Potentiation - (Maximisation)
Potion - (Potion)
Potion - (Potion)
poultice - (cataplasme)
Poverty - (Pauvreté)
Powder; dust - (Poudre, poussière)
Practice - (Exercer)
Prandial - (Prandial)

Preanesthesia - (Pré-anesthésie)

Precancerous - (Précancéreux)

Precarious - (Précaire)

Precipitation - (Précipitation)

Preclinical - (Pré-clinique)

Precordial - (Région précordiale)

Precursor - (Précurseur)

Prediabetic - (Pré-diabète)

Predisposition - (Prédisposition)

Pre-eclampsia - (Pré-éclampsie)

Pregnancy - (Enceinte)

Pregnant - (Enceinte)

Pregnant - (Enceinte)

Prejudicial; harmful - (Nuisible)

Preliminary - (Préliminaire)

Premature - (Prématuré)

Premature contractions - (Contractions précoces)

Premenstrual - (Prémenstruel)

Prenatal - (Prénatal)

Prenatal diagnosis - (Diagnostic prénatal)

Pre-operative care - (Soin pré-opératoire)

Preparatory studies - (Propédeutique)

Prepared - (Préparé (e))

Prepuce - (Prépuce)

Prescribe - (Prescrire)

Prescribe, to - (Prescrire)

Prescription - (Ordonnance)

Prescription - (Ordonnance, recette)

Prescription drug dependency - (Pharmacodépendance)

Prescription, medical - (Prescription médicale)

Present - (Présent)

Pressure - (Pression, tension)

Pressure gauge - (Manomètre)

Pressure, arterial - (Tension artérielle)

Pressure, osmotic - (Pression, tension osmotique)

Pressure, systolic blood - (Pression sanguine systolique)

Pretend, to - (Feindre, faire semblant)

Preterm - (Avant la fin)

Prevalence - (Prévalence)

Prevent, to - (Prévenir)

Prevention - (Prévention)

Prevention, health - (Prévention de santé)

Previous (or previa, after placenta) - (Préalable)

Priapism - (Priapisme)

Price - (Prix)

Primary - (Primaire)

Primary care - (Soins santé primaire)

Primigravida - (Enceinte pour la première fois)

Primipara - (Primipare)

Primitive - (Primitif)

Principal - (Principal)
Priority - (Prioritaire)
Privation; deprivation; loss -
(Privation)
Probability - (Probabilité)
Probe - (Sonde)
Problem - (Problème)
Procedure - (Procédure)
Process (in some sites may
mean medical chart) -
(Processus)
Proctalgia - (Proctalgie)
Proctitis - (Proctite, rectite)
Proctoscopy - (Rectoscopie)
Prodrome - (Prodrome)
Product - (Produit)
Profession - (Profession)
Professional - (Professionnel
(le))
Profit - (Bénéfice)
Profuse - (Abondant)
Progenitor; parent - (Parents)
Progesterone - (Progestérone)
Prognosis - (Pronostic)
Prognosis, bad - (Mauvais
pronostic)
Prognosticate - (Pronostiquer)
Program, health - (Programme
de santé)
Progressive - (Progressif (ive))
Prohibited - (Interdit (e))
Prolapse - (Prolapsus)
Proliferation - (Prolifération)
Prolonged - (Prolongé (e))
Promiscuity - (Promiscuité)
Promotion, health -

(Promotion de santé)
Prone; lying face down -
(Décubitus ventral)
Prophylaxis - (Prophylaxie)
Propranolol - (Propanolol)
Proptosis - (Exophtalmie)
Prospectus - (Prospectus)
Prostate - (Prostate)
Prostatic - (Prostatique)
Prostatism - (Prostatisme)
Prostatitis - (Prostatite)
Prosthesis - (Prothèse)
Prostration - (Prostration)
Protect, to - (Protéger)
Protein - (Protéine)
protein - (protéin)
Proteins, dietary - (Protéines
de la diète)
Proteinuria - (Protéinurie)
Proteolytic - (Protéolytique)
Protoplasm - (Protoplasme)
protozoa - (protozoaires)
Protozoan - (Protozoaire)
Protrusion - (Protrusion)
Proximal - (Proximal)
Pruritus - (Picotement,
démangeaison)
Pruritus - (Prurit)
Pseudopregnancy - (Pseudo
grossesse)
Pseudotumor - (Pseudo
tumeur)
Psoas - (Psoas)
Psoriasis - (Psoriasis)
Psoriasis - (Psoriasis)
Psychiatric - (Psychiatrique)

Psychiatrist - (Psychiatre)
Psychiatrist - (Psychiatrique)
Psychiatry - (Psychiatrie)
Psychological - (Psychologique)
Psychomotor - (Psychomoteur)
Psychopath - (Psychopathe)
Psychosis - (Psychose)
Psychosis - (Psychose)
Psychosocial - (Psychosocial)
Psychosomatic - (Psychosomatique)
Psychotherapy - (Psychothérapie)
Pterygium - (Ptérygion)
Ptosis - (Ptôsis, ptôse)
Puberty - (Puberté)
Pubis - (Pubis)
Public administration - (Administration publique)
Public assistance - (Assistance publique)
Public bathrooms - (Toilettes publiques)
Public health center - (Centre de santé publique)
Public water source - (Sources publiques d'eau)
Puerperal - (Puerpéral, (e, aux))
Pulmonary - (Pulmonaire)
Pulmonary fibrosis - (Fibrose pulmonaire)
Pulp; soft tissue - (Pulpe)

Pulsation - (Pulsation)
Pulse - (Pouls)
Pump - (Pompe)
Pump, to - (Pomper)
Puncture - (Ponction)
Puncture lumbar - (Ponction lombaire)
Pupa - (Pupe)
Pupil - (Pupille)
Pupil (of the eye) - (Pupille)
Puree - (Purée)
Purify, to - (Purifier)
Purpura; purple - (Pourpre)
Purpura; thrombocytopenic - (Purpura trombotique trombocitopénique)
Purulent - (Purulent(e))
Pus - (Pus)
pus - (pus)
Push, to - (Pousser)
Pustule - (Pustule)
Pustulous - (Pustuleux)
Put, to - (Placer, mettre)
Pyelonephritis - (Pyélonéphrite)
Pylorus - (Pylore)
Pyoderma - (Pyodermie)
Pyogenic - (Pyogène)
Pyonephritis - (Pyonéphrite)
Pyrexia - (Pyrexie)
Pyridoxine - (Pyridoxine)
Pyrogenic - (Pyrogène)
Pyrosis - (Pyrosis)
Pyuria - (Pyurie)

~ Q ~

Quadriceps - (Quadriceps)
Quadriplegia - (Quadriplégie)
Quadriplegia - (Tétraplégie)
Quadriplegic -
(Quadriplégique, tétraplégique)
Quadruplet - (Quadruplet)
Qualitative - (Qualitatif (ve))
Quality of life - (Qualité de vie)
Quality of medications -
(Qualité des médicaments)
Quantitative - (Quantitatif (ve))
Quarantine - (Quarentaine)
Question - (Question)
Question, to (ask a) - (Poser une question)
Question, to; interrogate - (Interroger)
Quinine - (Quinine)

~ R ~

Rabies; rage - (Rage)
Race - (Race)
Rachialgia - (Rachialgie)
Rachidian - (Rachidien)
Rachis; spinal column - (Rachis)
Rachitic; rickety - (Rachitique)
Racial - (Racial)
Radial - (Radial(le))

Radiant - (Radiant (e))
Radiation - (Radiation)
Radiation therapy - (Radiothérapie)
Radical - (Radical (e))
Radiculitis - (Radiculite)
Radiograph; X-ray - (Radiographie)
Radiologic protection - (Protection radiologique)
Radiologist - (Radiologue)
Radiology - (Radiologie)
Radiopaque - (Radiopaque)
Radiotransparent - (Radio transparent)
Rales; rasping breath - (Stertor, râle)
Ranula - (Ranule, grenouillette)
Rape, to - (Violer)
Raphe - (Raphé)
Rapid; fast - (Rapide, vite)
Rare - (Bizarre)
Rarefaction - (Raréfaction)
Rash - (Bouton de chaleur)
Rash, cutaneous eruption - (Rash, éruption cutanée)
Rate - (Taux)
Ration; serving - (Ration)
Rational - (Rationnel (le))
Reabsorb - (Réabsorber)
Reabsorption - (Réabsorption)
Reaction - (Réaction)
Reactivation - (Réactivation)
Reactive - (Réactif)
Reactivity - (Réactivité)

Reason - (Raison)
Recent - (Récent)
Receptor - (Récepteur)
Recession - (Récession)
Recessive - (Récessif)
Recessive characteristic -
(Héritage récessif,
héritagecytoplasmique)
Recommendable -
(Recommandable)
Recommendation -
(Recommandation)
Reconstitution -
(Reconstitution)
Record; file - (Record,
registre)
Recover, to - (Se rétablir)
Recovered - (Rétabli (e))
Recovery of health -
(Recouvrir la santé)
Rectal - (Rectal)
Rectally - (Voie rectale)
Rectification; correction -
(Rectification)
Rectocele - (Proctocèles)
Rectosigmoid - (Recto
sigmoïde)
Rectum - (Rectum)
rectum - (rectum)
Recuperation - (Récupération)
Recurrence; relapse -
(Récidive)
Recurrent - (Récurrent)
Red - (Rouge)
Red blood cell - (Globules
rouges)
Red blood cell count -
(Hématocrite)
Red blood cells - (Hématie)
Red Cross - (Croix Rouge)
Reddening - (Devenir rouge)
Redness; flushing - (Rougeur)
Reduction - (Réduction)
Refer, to - (Référer)
Reference - (Référence)
Referred - (Référé (e))
Reflection - (Réflection)
Reflex - (Réflexe)
Reflex; decortication -
(Réflexe de décortiquement)
Reflux - (Reflux)
Reflux gastroesophageal -
(Reflux gastro-œsophagien)
Refraction - (Réfraction)
Refractory - (Réfractaire)
Refusal - (Négation)
Regeneration - (Régénération)
Regimen - (Régime)
Regimen, therapeutic -
(Régime thérapeutique)
Regimen, weight loss -
(Régime d'amaigrissement)
Region; area - (Région)
Regional - (Régional)
Register, to - (Enregistrer)
Registry, medical - (Registre
médicale)
Regression - (Régression)
Regularly - (Régulièrement)
Regulation - (Régulation)

Regurgitation - (Régurgitation)
Rehabilitation - (Réhabilitation)
Rehabilitation center - (Centre de rééducation)
Rehydrate, to - (Réhydrater)
Rehydration - (Réhydratation)
Reinfection - (Reinfection)
Rejection - (Refus)
Relapse - (Rechute)
Related to food - (Alimentaire)
Relation; relationship - (Relation)
Relative, a - (Parents)
Relative, a; familiar - (Familier)
Relax oneself, to - (Se relaxer)
Relax, to - (Relaxer)
Relaxant - (Relaxant (e))
Release from hospital - (Autoriser la sortie de l'hôpital)
Relief - (Soulagement)
Relief, food - (Aide alimentaire)
Relieve, to; to aide - (Secourir)
Religion - (Religion)
Remedy, to; cure, to - (Remédier)
Remedy; cure - (Remède)
Remember, to - (Se rappeler)
Remission - (Rémission)
Remove all clothing; undress, to - (Déshabiller, dénuder)
Remove, to - (Enlever, retirer)

Remove, to - (Remuer)
Remove, to - (Retirer)
Renal - (Rénal)
Repeat, to - (Répéter)
repel - (repousser)
Replace, to - (Remplacer)
Replacement - (Reposition)
Reply; copy - (Réplique)
Report, to - (Reporter)
Repression - (Répression)
Reproduction - (Reproduction)
Resection - (Résection)
Reservoir - (Réservoir)
Residence, address - (Domicile)
Residual - (Résiduel (le))
Residual water - (Eau résiduelle)
Resin - (Résine)
Resistance - (Résistance)
Resistance, antibiotic - (Résistance aux antibiotiques)
Resistance, medication - (Résistance aux médicaments)
Resistant - (Résistant (e))
resistant - (résistant)
Resonance - (Résonance)
Resources, health - (Ressources de santé)
Respiration - (Respiration)
Respiratory - (Respiratoire)
Respiratory rate - (Fréquence respiratoire)
Respiratory system - (Appareil respiratoire)
Response; answer -

(Réponse)
Responsible - (Responsable)
Rest - (Repos)
Rest bed - (Repos au lit)
Rest period - (Période de repos)
Rest, a - (Repos)
Rest, to - (Reposer)
Result - (Résultat)
Resuscitate, to - (Réanimer)
Resuscitate, to - (Ressusciter)
Resuscitation - (Réanimation)
Resuscitation - (Ressuscitation)
Retardation, mental - (Oligophrénie)
Retarded, mentally - (Oligophrène)
Retention - (Rétention)
Retention, Fluid - (Rétention de liquides)
reticulum - (réticulum)
Retina - (Rétine)
retina - (rétine)
Retinal ablation - (Ablation de la rétine)
Retinopathy - (Rétinopathie)
Retraction - (Rétraction)
Retroflexion - (Rétroflexion)
Retrograde - (Rétrograde)
Retrolingual - (Rétro lingual)
Retroocular - (Retro oculaire)
Retroperitoneal - (Rétro périnée)
Retrospective - (Rétrospectif

(ve))
Return, to - (Retourner)
Reverse, to - (Intervertir)
Reversible - (Réversible)
Review; magazine - (Revue)
Revive, to - (Revivre)
Revulsive - (Révulsif (ive))
Rhabdomyolysis - (Rhabdomyolyse)
Rheumatic fever - (Fière rhumatismale)
Rheumatism - (Rhumatisme)
Rheumatism - (Rhumatisme)
Rheumatoid - (Rhumatoïde)
Rhinitis - (Rhinite)
Rhinitis, allergic - (Rhinite allergique)
Rhinorrhea - (Rhinorrhée)
Rhythm - (Rythme)
Rhythm, cardiac - (Rythme cardiaque)
Rhythmic - (Rythmique)
Rib - (Côte)
Riboflavin - (Riboflavine)
Rickets; rachitis - (Rachitisme)
rickettsia - (rickettsies)
Rifampin - (Rifampicine)
Right - (Droit(e))
Right hand - (Main droite)
Rigidity; stiffness - (Rigidité)
Ring finger - (Annulaire)
Ring finger - (Annulaire)
Risk - (Risque)
Risk factor - (Facteur de risque)

Rodent control - (Contrôle de rongeurs)
Roof - (Toiture)
Room - (Chambre)
Room operating (surgical) - (Salle d´opération)
Room, delivery - (Salle d'accouchement)
Room, operating - (Salon d'opération)
Room, recovery - (Salle de récupération)
Room, waiting - (Salle d'attente)
Root - (Racine)
Root (of a tooth) - (Chicot)
Rotation - (Rotation)
Rotten - (Pourri(e))
Rough - (Rugueux)
Roughness - (Caractère de ce qui est rugueux)
Round - (Rond (e))
roundworms - (ascaris)
Rub, to - (Frotter)
Rub; friction - (Frottement)
Rubella - (Rougeole)
rumen - (rumen)
ruminant - (ruminants)
ruminate - (ruminer)
Rupture - (Rupture)

~ S ~

Sac - (Sac)
Saccharine - (Saccharine)

Sacroilitis - (Inflammation des jointures)
Sacrolumbar - (Sacro lombaire)
Safe (salubrious) - (Salubre)
Sagittal - (Sagittal)
Salicylate - (Salicylate)
Salicylic acid - (Acide salicylique)
Salicylism (salicylate toxicity) - (Salicylisme)
Saliva - (Salive)
saliva - (salive)
Salivary glands - (Glandes salivaires)
Salmonella - (Salmonelle)
Salpingitis - (Salpingite)
Salt - (Sel)
Salty - (Salé)
Sample - (Echantillon)
Sanitary - (Sanitaire)
Saphenous - (Saphène)
Saprophyte - (Saprophyte)
sarcoid - (sarcoïde)
Sarcoma - (Sarcome)
Sarcoma, kaposi's - (Sarcome de Kaposi)
Saturation - (Saturation)
Saturation, oxygen - (Saturation d'oxygène)
Save, to - (Sauver)
Scab - (Croûte)
scab - (tavelure)
Scabicide - (Scabicide)
Scabies - (Gale)
Scabies - (Gale)

Scabies - (Scabiose, gale)
Scale (for weighing) [as noun];
weighs [verb] - (Balance)
Scalpel - (Scalpel, bistouri)
Scaly; flaky - (Écailleux(se))
Scan; tracking - (Dépister)
Scapel - (Bistouri)
Scapula - (Omoplate)
Scapula; shoulder blade - (Os
scapulaire)
Scar - (Cicatrice)
Scar formation -
(Cicatrisation)
Scarlet fever - (Scarlatine)
Schizophrenia -
(Schizophrénie)
Sciatica - (Sciatique)
Science - (Science)
Scissors - (Ciseaux)
Sclerosis - (Sclérose)
Sclerotic - (Sclérotique)
Scoliosis - (Scoliose)
Scratch - (Égratignure)
Scratch oneself, to - (Se
gratter)
Scratch, to - (Gratter)
Screen - (Écran)
Scrotum - (Scrotum)
scrotum - (scrotum)
Scurvy - (Scorbut)
Seal, to - (Obturer)
Search and rescue -
(Opération de sauvetage)
Sea-sick, dizzy - (Atteint du
mal de mer)

Seated; sitting (adj) -
(Assis(se))
Seborrhea - (Séborrhée)
Seborrheic dermatitis -
(Dermatite séborique)
Secondary - (Secondaire)
Secondary care - (Soins
secondaires)
Secretary - (Secrétariat)
Secretion - (Sécrétion)
Sedate, to - (Apaiser, Calmer)
Sedated - (Sous l'effet d'un
sédatif)
Sedative - (Anxiolytique)
Sedative - (Sédatif)
Sedentary - (Sédentaire)
Sediment - (Sédiment)
Sedimentation -
(Sédimentation)
See, to - (Voir)
Segment - (Segment)
Segregation - (Ségrégation)
Select, to - (Sélectionner)
Selection - (Sélection)
Selective - (Sélectif (ve))
Self-Care - (Auto soins, se
soigner soimême)
Self-Medication -
(Automédication)
Semen - (Liquide séminal,
sperme)
semen - (sperme)
Semiotic - (Sémiotique)
Senile - (Sénile)
Senility - (Sénilité)

Senior citizen - (Personne âgée)
Sensation - (Sensation)
Sense (5 senses or instinct) - (Sens)
Sensible - (Sensible)
Sensitivity - (Sensibilité)
Sensitization - (Sensibilisation)
Sensory - (Sensoriel (le))
Sensual - (Sensuel)
Separation - (Séparation)
Sepsis - (Sepsis, infection)
Septic - (Septique)
septicaemia - (septicémie)
Septicemia - (Septicémie)
Septum - (Cloison)
Septum - (Cloison nasale, septum nasal)
Septum, Nasal - (Os du nez)
Sequelae - (Séquelles)
Sequential - (En séquence)
Serious - (Grave)
Serious - (Sérieux(se))
Serious disease - (Maladie grave)
Seroconversion - (Développement d'anticorpsdétectables)
Serological - (Sérologique)
Serology - (Sérologie)
Seronegative - (Séronégatif (ive))
Seropositive - (Séropositif (ive))
Serotype - (Sérotype)
Serovigilance - (Sérovigilance)

Serum - (Sérum)
Sex; intercourse - (Sexe)
Sexual abuse - (Abus sexuel)
Sexual chromosome - (Chromosome sexuel)
Sexual education - (Education sexuelle)
Sexual harassment - (Harcèlement sexuel)
Sexuality - (Sexualité)
Sexually Transmitted Infection; STI - (Maladies sexuellement transmissibles MST)
shake, to - (Agiter)
Sheath - (Gaine)
Shigella - (Shigella)
Shigellosis - (Shigellose)
Shipping - (Envoi)
Shirt - (Chemise)
Shiver - (Frisson)
Shock, to - (Emouvoir, émotionner)
Shorten, to - (Écourter)
Shoulder - (Epaule)
Shout - (Cris)
Sialogogues - (Sialagogue)
Sick - (Malade)
Sick with a cold - (Enrhumé)
Sickle cell - (Drépanocyte)
Sickle cell anemia - (Anémie falciforme)
Sickle cell disease - (Drépanocytose)
Sickness - (Maladie)
Siderosis - (Sidéropénie)
Sig (dosing plan, as in

prescription) - (Posologie)
Sigmoid; sigmoidal -
(Sigmoïde)
Sign - (Signe)
Signal - (Signal)
Signature - (Signature)
Significant - (Significatif)
Similar - (Similaire)
Simulated - (Simulé (e))
Single-cell - (Unicellulaire)
Sinovitis - (Synovite)
Sinus; breast - (Sein)
Sinuses paranasal - (Sinus
nasaux)
Sinusitis - (Sinusite)
Situation - (Situation)
Sixth - (Sixième)
Size - (Grandeur)
Size (as in clothing); waist -
(Taille)
Skeleton - (Squelette)
Skin - (Peau)
Skin - (Peau)
Skin irritation - (Dermatite
irritante)
Skin, cracked - (Peau gercée)
Sleep inducing - (Qui endort)
Sleep, to - (Dormir)
Sleep; dream - (Rêve)
Sleeping pill - (Somnifère)
Sleepwalking -
(Somnambulisme)
Slimming; weight loss -
(Amaigrissement)
Slit; crack; split - (Incision)

Slowly - (Doucement)
Small - (Petit (e))
Small - (Tout petit, minuscule)
Small pox - (Variole)
Smear - (Frottis)
Smell, sense of - (Odorat)
Smell, to - (Sentir)
Smile - (Sourire)
Smoke, to - (Fumer)
Smoker - (Fumeur)
Smooth - (Lisse)
Smooth - (Suave, doux,
douce)
Snake - (Serpent)
Sneeze - (Éternuement)
Sneeze, to - (Éternuer)
Soap - (Savon)
Social conditions - (Conditions
sociales)
Social wellbeing - (Bien-être
social)
Social worker - (Travailleur
social)
Society - (Société)
Soft; bland - (Mou/Molle)
Soften, to - (Ramollir)
Softening - (Amollissement)
Sole; bottom of the foot -
(Plante du pied)
Solid - (Solide)
Soluble - (Soluble)
Solution - (Solution)
Solution, gargling - (Solution
pour faire des gargarismes)
Solution, saline - (Solution

saline)
Solvent - (Dissolvant)
Soma - (Soma)
Somatic - (Somatique)
Somatization - (Somatisation)
Somnolence - (Somnolence)
Son - (Fils)
Soon - (Prompt)
Soporific - (Soporifique)
Sore throat - (Mal de gorge)
Sound - (Son)
Soup; broth - (Bouillon)
Sour - (Aigre)
sour stomach - (Acidité)
Source - (Source)
Source of the illness - (Source de la maladie)
Soy - (Soya, Soja)
Spasm - (Spasme)
Spastic - (Spasmodique)
Spastic - (Spastique)
Spasticity - (Spasticité)
Speak, to - (Parler)
Specialist - (Spécialiste)
Species - (Espèce)
Specific - (Spécifique)
Spectrum - (Spectre)
Speculum - (Spéculum)
Sperm - (Sperme)
sperm - (sperme)
spermatic cord - (cordon spermatique)
Spermatozoid - (Spermatozoïde)
Spermicide - (Spermicide)
Sphenoid - (Sphénoïde)

Sphincter - (Sphincter)
Sphincterectomy - (Sphinctérectomie)
Spina bifida - (Épine bifide)
Spinal cord - (Moelle épinière)
Spine - (Épine dorsale)
Spirit - (Esprit)
Spleen - (Rate)
spleen - (rate)
Spondylitis - (Spondylite)
Sporadic - (Sporadique)
spore - (spores)
Sport - (Sport)
Spouse - (Époux/ Épouse)
Spouse - (mari)
Sprain - (Entorse)
Sprain - (Entorse)
Sprained - (Tordu (e))
spray - (Aérosol)
Spring (the season) - (Printemps)
Sprue - (Sprue)
Spur - (Éperon sous-calcanéen)
Sputum - (Crachat)
Squatting - (Accroupi)
Stab wound - (Blessure par arme blanche)
Stabbing pain; shooting pain - (Élancement)
Stain; blemish - (Tache)
Staphylococcemia - (Staphylococcie)
Staphylococcus - (Staphylocoque)
Starch - (Amidon)

Starving - (Affamé (e))
State - (État)
State of health - (État de santé)
Statistic - (Statistique)
Stature - (Stature)
Steatorrhoea - (Excès de gras dans les matières fécales)
Stenosis - (Sténose)
Sterile - (Stérile)
sterile - (stérile)
sterilise - (stériliser)
Sterility - (Stérilité)
Sterilization - (Stérilisation)
Sternal angle; manubriosternal joint - (Manivelle du sternum)
Sternocleidomastoid - (Sterno-cléido-mastoïdien,muscle au cou)
Sternum - (Sternum)
Stethoscope - (Stéthoscope)
Stiffen - (Ankyloser)
Stigma - (Stigmate)
Stimulant - (Stimulant)
Stimulation - (Stimulation)
Stimulus - (Stimulus)
Stink; foul odor - (Puer, odeur fétide)
Stomach - (Estomac)
stomach - (estomac)
Stomach, sick to the - (Mal a' l'estomac)
Stomatitis - (Stomatite)
Stomatologist; dentist - (Dentiste, stomatologue)

Stone - (Calcul, pierre)
Stone - (Pierre, caillou)
Stone, urinary - (Formation de calcul dans l'urètre)
Stones, kidney; renal calculi - (Pierres aux reins)
Stop, to - (Arrêter)
Strabismus - (Strabisme)
Strabismus; crossed eyes - (Loucher, strabisme)
Strange; foreign - (Bizarre, rare)
Strawberry - (Fraise)
Streak; line - (Ligne)
Strength; potency - (Puissance)
Streptococcus - (Streptocoque)
Streptococcus - (Streptocoque)
Streptokinase - (Streptokinase)
Streptomycin - (Streptomycine)
Stress - (Stress)
stress - (le stress)
Stretcher - (Brancard)
Stria; stretch mark - (Vergeture)
Strokes, brush - (Badigeonnage)
Strongyloidiasis - (Strongyloïdose)
Structure - (Structure)
Stump - (Moignon)

Stupor - (Stupeur)
Stutterer - (Bègue)
Stye - (Orgelet)
Sub-acute - (Subaigu)
Subcapsular - (Sous-capsulaire)
Sub-clinical - (Sous-clinique)
Subcostal - (Sous-cotes)
Subcutaneous - (Sous-cutanée)
Sub-dural - (Subdural (le))
Subdural hematoma - (Hématome sud dural)
Subgroup - (Sous- groupe)
Subjective - (Subjectif (ive))
Sublingual - (Sublingual)
Submandibular - (Sous-mandibulaire)
Submucosa - (Sous-muqueuse)
Subphrenic - (Sous-phrénique)
Subscapular - (Subscapulaire)
Substance - (Substance)
Substitute, breastmilk - (Substitut du lait maternel)
Substitution; replacement - (Substitution, remplacement)
Substitutions; replacement - (Substitut, remplaçant)
Substrate - (Substrat)
Suck, to - (Sucer)
Suck, to - (Sucer)
Suckle, to - (Téter)
Suction - (Succion)
Suction cup - (Ventouse)

Sudden - (Soudain)
Sudden - (Subitement)
Sudden disease - (Maladie soudaine)
Suffer, to - (Souffrir)
Suffering - (Agonie)
Suffering - (Souffrance)
Sufficient - (Suffisant (e))
Sugar - (Sucre)
Suggest, to - (Suggérer)
Suicide - (Suicide)
Summarize, to - (Résumer)
Summary - (Résumé)
Summer - (Été)
Sun - (Soleil)
Superciliary - (Sourcilière)
Superficial - (Superficielle)
Super-infection - (Super infection)
Superior - (Supérieur)
Superstition - (Superstition)
Supervise, to - (Superviser)
Supine; lying face up - (Décubitus dorsal)
Supper - (Repas)
Supperate; ooze; discharge, to - (Suppurer)
Supperation; discharge - (Suppuration)
Supplement - (Supplément)
supplement - (supplément)
Supplement, vitamin - (Supplément vitaminique)
Supply, to - (Approvisionner, ravitailler)
Suppository - (Suppositoire)

Suppression - (Suppression)
Supraclavicular - (Supra claviculaire)
Supraventricular - (Supra ventriculaire)
Supraventricular arrhythmia - (Arythmie supra ventriculaire)
Sure - (Sûr (e))
Surgeon - (Chirurgien)
Surgery - (Chirurgie)
Surgical - (Chirurgical (e))
Surgical gloves - (Gants chirurgicaux)
Surplus - (Reste)
Surrounding; environment of - (Entourage, environnement)
Surveillance, health - (Vigilance, surveillance sanitaire)
Survive, to - (Survivre)
Survivor - (Survivant)
Susceptible - (Susceptible)
Suspension - (Suspension)
Suttering; stammering - (Bégayer)
Suture - (Suture)
suture - (suture)
Suture; stitch, to - (Suturer)
Swallow - (Avaler)
Swallowing - (Déglutition)
Sweat - (Sueur, transpiration)
Sweat, to - (Suer, transpirer)
Sweats, night - (Sueurs nocturnes)
Sweet - (Doux(ce))

Sweet - (Saccharose)
Swell, to - (Enfler)
Swell, to - (Tuméfier)
Swelling - (Épaississement, engraisser)
Swelling - (Gonflement)
Swelling - (Tuméfaction)
Swollen - (Enflé (e))
Symmetric - (Symétrique)
Sympathomimetic - (Sympatico- mimétique)
Symptom - (Symptôme)
Symptom, late - (Symptôme retardé)
Symptom, simulated - (Symptômes simulés)
Symptomatic - (Symptomatique)
Symptomatology - (Symptomatologie)
Synapse - (Synapse)
Syncope - (Syncope)
Syncronous - (Synchronique)
Syndrome - (Syndrome)
Syndrome, Down - (Syndrome de Down)
Syndrome, nephrotic - (Syndrome néphrétique)
Synergistic - (Synergique)
Synergy - (Synergie)
Synonymous - (Synonyme)
Synovial - (Synovial)
Synovial effusion - (Épanchement liquide synovial)
Synthesis - (Synthèse)

Syphilis - (Syphilis)
Syphilitic - (Atteint de syphilis)
Syphilitic - (Syphilitique,
luétique)
Syringe - (Seringue)
Syrup - (Sirop)
System, Health - (Système de
santé)
System, life support -
(Système de maintien de la
vie)
Systematic - (Systématique)
Systemic - (Systémique)
Systole - (Systole)
Systolic - (Systolique)

~ T ~

Table; Plank - (Tableau)
Tablet - (Comprimé)
Taboo - (Tabou)
Tachyarrhythmia -
(Tachyarythmie)
Tachycardia - (Tachycardie)
Tachypnea - (Tachypnée)
Take - (Boire, prendre,
prélever)
Talc - (Poudre)
Tamponage -
(Tamponnement)
Tank, septic - (Fosse septique)
Tannin - (Tannin)
Tapeworm - (Cestoïde)
tapeworm - (ténia)
Tarsus - (Tarse)

Tartar - (Tartre, saburre)
Taste - (Goût)
Taste - (Saveur)
Tea - (Thé)
Teach, to; show, to -
(Montrer)
Teacher - (Maître / Maîtresse)
Team - (Équipe)
Tear - (Déchirement)
Tear - (Larme)
Technician - (Technique)
Technology - (Technologie)
Teleangiectasia -
(Télangiectasie)
Teleconference -
(Téléconférence)
Temperature - (Température)
Temperature; fever -
(Température élevée, fièvre)
Temple - (Tempe)
Tendinitis - (Tendinite)
Tendon - (Tendon)
tendon - (tendon)
Tendon, Achilles - (Tendon
d'Achille)
Tenesmus - (Ténesme)
Tenia - (Ténia, ver solitaire)
Tenosynovitis - (Ténosynovite)
Tense - (Tendu (e))
Tension; pressure - (Tension)
Tenth - (Dixième)
Teratogenic - (Tératogénique)
Teratogenic agent - (Agent
tératogène)
Teratogeny - (Tératogène)
Teratoma - (Tératome)

Terminal - (Terminal)
Terminal cancer - (Cancer terminal)
Terminal care - (Soin terminal)
Terminal disease - (Maladie terminale)
Terror - (Terreur)
Tertiary care - (Soins tertiaires)
Test - (Test, examen)
Test; essay - (Essai, pratique, test)
Test; proof; analysis - (Test, analyse)
Testicle - (Testicule)
testicles - (testicules)
Testicular - (Testiculaire)
Testing; study - (Culture)
Testosterone - (Testostérone)
Tetanus - (Tétanos)
Tetany - (Tétanie)
Tetracycline - (Tétracycline)
Tetralogy of fallot - (Tétralogie de Fallot)
Texture - (Texture)
Thalamus - (Thalamus)
Thalassemia - (Thalassémie)
Theophylline - (Théophylline)
Theoretical - (Théorique)
Therapeutic - (Thérapeutique)
Therapeutic diet - (Alimentation thérapeutique)
Therapy - (Thérapie)
Therefore - (Donc)
Thermal - (Thermique)

Thermometer - (Thermomètre)
Thermoregulation - (Thermorégulation)
Thiabendazole - (Thiabendazole)
Thiamin - (Thiamine)
Thick - (Gros(se), épais(se))
Thickness - (Grosseur)
Thigh - (Cuisse)
Thin - (Mince)
Think, to - (Penser)
Third - (Troisième)
third eyelid - (troisième paupière)
Thirst - (Soif)
Thoracic - (Thoracique)
Thoracic cage - (Cage thoracique)
Thoraco-abdominal - (Thoraco-abdominal)
Thorax; Chest - (Thorax)
Threat - (Menace)
Three times a day, TID - (Trois fois par jour)
Throat - (Gorge)
Thrombembolism - (Thromboembolie)
Thrombembolytic - (Thrombolytique)
Thrombocytopenia - (Thrombopénie)
Thrombophlebitis - (Thrombophlébite)
Thrombosis - (Thrombose)

Thrombus - (Thrombus, caillot sanguin)
Throw - (Tirer)
Thumb - (Pouce)
Thumb - (Pouce)
Thymus - (Thymus)
Thyroid - (Thyroïde)
thyroid gland   - (glande thyroïde)
Thyroiditis - (Thyroïdites)
Tibia - (Tibia)
Tibial - (Tibial (le))
Tic - (Tic)
Tick - (Tique)
Timbre - (Timbre)
Time - (Temps)
Timolol - (Timolol)
Tinea - (Teigne)
Tinnitus - (Acouphène)
Tinnitus - (Acouphène)
Tired - (Fatigué(e))
Tissue - (Tissu)
Tissue, subcutaneous - (Tissu cutané)
Tissue-like - (Tissulaire)
Title; degree - (Diplôme)
Tobacco - (Tabac, cigare)
Tobacco poisoning - (Tabagisme)
Today - (Aujourd'hui)
Toes - (Orteils)
Tolerance - (Tolérance)
Tolerance to the drug - (Tolérance au médicament)
Tolerate - (Tolérer)
Tomography - (Tomographie)

Tomorrow - (Demain)
Tone - (Tonus)
Tongue - (Langue)
Tonic - (Tonique)
Tonic-clonic - (Spasme musculaire tonicoclonique)
Tonsilitis - (Amygdalite)
Tonsillar - (Amygdale)
Tonsillectomy - (Amygdalectomie)
Tonsillectomy - (Amygdalectomie)
Tonsillitis - (Amygdalite)
Tonsils - (Amygdales)
Tooth - (Dent)
Toothache - (Mal aux dents)
Toothache - (Odontalgie)
Toothbrush - (Brosse à dents)
Toothpaste - (Dentifrice)
Topical application - (Application topique)
Topical; for external use - (Topique)
Torpor - (Sommeil profond)
Torsion - (Torsion)
Torso - (Torse)
Torticollis - (Torticolis)
Total - (Total)
Touch - (Tact)
Touch - (Toucher)
Toxemia - (Toxémie)
Toxic - (Toxique)
Toxic effect - (Effet toxique)
Toxicity - (Toxicité)
Toxin - (Toxine)
Toxin, tetanus - (Toxine

tétanique)
Toxoid - (Toxoïde)
Toxoplasmosis -
(Toxoplasmose)
Trachea - (trachée)
trachea - (La trachée)
Tracheal - (Trachéal)
Tracheitis - (Trachéite)
Tracheotomy; tracheostomy -
(Trachéotomie)
Trachoma - (Trachome)
Tract - (Tractus)
Tranquil; calm - (Tranquille)
Tranquilizer - (Tranquillisant)
Transaminase -
(Transaminase)
Transferral - (Transfert)
Transform - (Transformer)
Transfuse - (Faire une
transfusion)
Transfusion - (Transfusion)
Transfusion, blood -
(Transfusion sanguine)
Transient - (Transitoire)
Transient ischemic attack -
(Crise ischémique transitoire)
Transit accidents - (Accident
de la route)
Translation - (Traduction)
Translocation - (Translocation)
Transmissible - (Transmissible)
Transmissible diseases -
(Maladies transmissibles)
Transmission - (Transmission)
Transmit - (Transmettre)

Transmitter - (Transmetteur
(euse))
Transplant - (Transplantation,
greffe)
Transvaginal - (Transvaginale)
Trash - (Ordures, déchets,
résidus)
Trashcan - (Poubelle)
Trauma - (Trauma)
Trauma, Birth - (Traumatisme
obstétricien)
Traumatic - (Traumatique)
Traumatism - (Traumatisme)
Treat - (Traiter)
Treatment - (Guérison)
Treatment - (Traitement)
Treatment room - (Chambre
de soins)
Treatment, cheaper alternative
- (Traitement alternatif moins
cher)
Treatment, maintenance -
(Traitement de maintient)
Treatment, outpatient -
(Traitement ambulatoire)
Treatment, preventive -
(Traitement préventif)
Treatment, water -
(Traitement de l'eau)
Tremor - (Tremblement)
Tremulous - (Tremblant)
Trend - (Tendance)
Trepanation - (Trépanation)
Treponema pallidum -
(Tréponème pâle)

Triad - (Triade)
Triceps - (Triceps)
Tricyclic - (Tricyclique)
Trimester - (Trimestre)
Triplets - (Triplets)
Trismus - (Trismus, tétanos)
trochar and cannula   - (trocart et la canule)
Trophic - (Trophique)
Trousers; pants - (Pantalon)
Trunk - (Tronc)
Truth - (Vérité)
Try, to; try out, to; prove, to - (Prouver, essayer)
Tube - (Trompe)
Tube - (Tube)
Tube, fallopian - (Trompe de Fallope)
Tube, uterine - (Trompe utérine)
Tuber - (Tubercule)
Tuberculin - (Tuberculine)
Tuberculosis - (Tuberculose)
Tuberculous - (Tuberculeux)
Tuberosity - (Tubérosité)
Tuboovarian - (Relatif aux trompes de Fallopeet l'ovaire)
Tubular - (Tubulaire)
Tumescent - (Turgide)
Tumor - (Néoplasie)
Tumor - (Tumeur)
Tumor, benign/malignant - (Tumeur bénigne/maligne)
Tumor, Primary - (Tumeur primaire)
Tumor, Secondary - (Tumeur secondaire)
Tumoral - (Tumoral (e))
tumour   - (Une croissance tumorale)
Turn red, to - (Rougir)
Tweezers; forceps; clamps - (Pince)
Twice a day - (Deux fois par jour)
Twin - (Jumeau)
Twins - (Jumeaux, Jumelles)
twitch - (twitch)
Typhoid - (Typhoïde)
Typhoid fever - (Fièvre typhoïde)
Typhus - (Typhus)
Typical - (Typique)

~ U ~

ulcer - (ulcère)
Ulcer, decubitus - (Ulcère de décubitus, plaiede lit)
Ulcer, gastric - (Ulcère)
Ulcer, peptic - (Ulcère peptique)
Ulcer; sore - (Plaie)
Ulceration - (Ulcération)
Ulcerous - (Ulcéreux (se))
Ulcers - (Ulcères)
Ulna - (Cubitus)
Ultrasonography - (Ultrasonographie)
Ultrasound - (Écographie)
Ultrasound, diagnostic -

(Écographie diagnostique)
Umbilical - (Ombilical)
Umbilical cord - (Cordon ombilical)
umbilical cord - (cordon ombilical)
Unbearable; intolerable - (Insupportable)
Uncle - (Oncle)
Unconscious - (Inconscient)
uncoordinated - (non coordonnée)
Uncover - (Ouvrir, découvrir)
Underdeveloped - (Sous-développé (e))
Underground water - (Eau de source)
Underneath - (Dessous)
Undernourishment - (Sous-alimentation)
Understand - (Comprendre)
Undifferentiated - (Sans différence)
Undress oneself - (Dévêtir)
uneasy - (Agité(e))
Unharmed - (Indemne)
Unhygienic - (Antihygiénique)
UNICEF - (UNICEF)
Uniform - (Uniforme)
Uninhibited - (Desinhibation)
Union - (Union)
Unique - (Unique)
United - (Uni (e))
Universal - (Universel)
University - (Université)

Unnecessary - (Non nécessaire)
Unperforated - (Imperforé(e))
Unspecific - (Non spécifique)
Unstable - (Instable)
Until - (Jusqu'a)
Unwanted - (Indésirable)
Upper limb - (Extrémité supérieure)
Uraemia - (Urémie)
Urea - (Urée)
Ureter - (Urètre)
Urethra - (Urètre)
Urethritis - (Urétrite)
Urge; straining; push - (Épreinte)
Urgent - (Urgent)
Urgent Care - (Soins d'urgence)
Uric - (Urique)
Uric acid - (Acide urique)
Urinal - (Pot de nuit)
Urinary - (Urinaire)
Urinary bladder - (Vessie urinaire)
urinate - (uriner)
Urinate, to - (Uriner)
Urine - (Urine)
Urogenital - (Génito-urinaire)
Urography - (Urographie)
Urology - (Urologie)
Urosepsis - (Urétrite)
Use (n.) - (Usage)
Use (v.) - (User)
Use up - (Usure, usage)

Uterocervical - (Utéro- cervical (e))
uterus - (utérus)
Uterus; womb - (Utérus)
Uveitis - (Uvéite)
Uvula - (Uvule)

~ V ~

Vaccinated - (Vacciné (e))
Vaccination - (Vaccination)
Vaccination campaign - (Campagne de vaccination)
Vaccine - (Vaccin)
vaccine - (vaccin)
Vagal; vagus nerve, of the - (Vagal)
Vagina - (Vagin)
vagina - (vagin)
Vaginal - (Vaginal)
Vaginal smear - (Frottis vaginal)
Vaginitis - (Vaginite)
Vaginosis - (Vaginose)
Vaginosis, bacterial - (Vaginose bactérienne)
Vagolytic - (Vagolytique)
Vagotonia - (Vagotomie)
Vagus (nerve); vague; vagrant - (Vague)
Validity - (Validité)
Valve - (Valve)
Valve - (Valvule)
Valve, bicuspid - (Valvule mitrale)

Valve, tricuspid - (Valvule tricuspide)
Valves, venous - (Valvules veineuses)
Valvular - (Valvulaire)
Valvulitis - (Inflammation d'une valvule)
Valvuloplasty - (Réparation d'une valvule cardiaque)
Valvulotomy - (Valvulotomie)
Vaporization - (Vaporisation)
Vaporizer - (Vaporisateur)
Variability - (Variabilité)
Variation - (Variation)
Varicocele - (Varicocèle)
Varicose - (Variqueux (euse))
Varicose veins - (Varices)
Varied - (Varié(e))
Variety - (Variété)
Various; several - (Plusieurs)
Vary, to; change, to - (Varier)
Vascular - (Vasculaire)
Vasculitis - (Vasculite)
Vasectomy - (Vasectomie)
Vaseline - (Vaseline)
Vasoactive - (Vaisseau-actif)
Vasoconstriction - (Vasoconstriction)
Vasoconstrictor - (Vasoconstricteur)
Vasodilatation - (Vasodilatation)
Vasodilator - (Vasodilatateur)
Vasomotor - (Vasomoteur)
Vasopressor - (Vasopresseur)
Vector - (Vecteur)

Vegetable - (Légume)
Vegetarian - (Végétarien)
Vegetative state - (État végétatif)
Vehicle - (Véhicule)
Vein - (Veine)
vein - (veine)
Vein, engorged - (Veine ingurgitée)
Veins - (veines)
Venereal - (Vénérien)
Venereal disease - (Maladie vénérienne)
Ventilation - (Ventilation)
Ventilation, artificial - (Ventilation artificielle)
Ventilator; fan - (Ventilateur)
Ventral - (Ventral)
Ventricle - (Ventricule)
Ventricular - (Ventriculaire)
Ventricular arrhythmia - (Arythmie ventriculaire)
Ventricular failure - (Défaillance ventriculaire)
Ventricular fibrillation - (Fibrillation ventriculaire)
Venule - (Veinule)
Verbosity - (Verbosité)
Vermicide - (Vermicide)
Vermiform - (vermiforme)
Vermis - (Vermisseau)
Vertebrae - (Vertèbre)
Vertebral Column - (Colonne vertébrale)
Vertebrocostal - (Vertébro-costal)
Vertex - (Vertex)
Vertigo - (Vertige)
Vertigo; sea sickness - (Vertige)
Very - (Très)
Vesical - (Biliaire)
Vesicle; bladder - (Vésicule)
Vessel - (Verre, vaisseau)
vessel - (navire)
Vessel, blood - (Vaisseau sanguin)
Vial - (Fiole, ampoule)
Vial; blister - (Ampoule)
Vibrio; vibrion - (Vibrion)
Vice - (Vice)
Villi - (Villosité)
Violence - (Violence)
Viral - (Virale)
Viral illness - (Virosite)
Viremia - (Virémie)
Virgin - (Vierge)
Virile - (Virilité)
Virilization; masculinization - (Devenir virile)
Virulent - (Virulent (e))
Virus - (Virus)
virus - (virus)
Visceral - (Viscéral e))
Viscosity - (Viscosité)
Viscous - (Visqueux)
Visible - (Visible)
Vision - (Vision)
Vision - (Vue)
Visit - (Visite)

Visit, medical - (Visite médicale)

Visiting hours - (Heure de visite)

Visual - (Visuel (le))

Visual acuity - (Acuité visuelle)

Visual field - (Champ visuel)

Vital capacity - (Capacité vitale)

Vitamin - (Vitamine)

Vitamin deficiency - (Déficience vitaminique)

vitamins - (vitamines)

Vitiligo - (Vitiligo)

Vitreous - (Vitreux (euse))

Vocal cords - (Cordes vocales)

Voice - (Voix)

Volume - (Volume)

Volunteer - (Bénévole)

Vomer bone - (Vomer)

Vomit - (Vomi, vomissement)

Vomit, to - (Vomir)

Vomiting, emesis - (Vomissement)

Voraciousness - (Voracité)

Vulnerable - (Vulnérable)

Vulva - (Vulve)

vulva - (vulve)

Vulvar - (Vulvaire)

Vulvitis - (Vulvite)

Vulvo vaginitis - (Vulvo-vaginite)

~ W ~

Waist - (Taille)

Wakefulness - (État de veille, surveillance)

Walk, to - (Marcher)

Walk, to; to ride - (Marcher, se promener)

Wall - (Mur)

Want, to - (Vouloir)

Warehouse - (Dépotoir, dépôt)

Warfarin (a blood thinner medication) - (Warfarine (médicament) mauvaise eau de vie)

Wart - (Verrue)

Wasp - (Guêpe)

Waste - (Déchet)

Water - (Eau)

Water (Air) contamination; pollution - (Contamination de l'eau (del'air))

Water quality - (Qualité de l'eau)

Water soluble - (Hydrosoluble)

Water supply - (Approvisionnement d'eau)

Watery; aqueous - (Aqueux(se))

Wave - (Onde)

Weak - (Faible)

Weakness - (Faiblesse, débilité)

wean - (sevrer)

Wean, to - (Sevrer)

Weaning - (Sevrage)

Web; internet - (WEB)

Week - (Semaine)

Weekly - (Hebdomadaire)
Weight - (Poids)
Weight, birth - (Poids à la naissance)
Weight, body - (Poids corporel)
Welcome - (Bienvenu(e))
Well (noun), artesian - (Puits artésien)
Wellbeing - (Bien-être)
Wet; damp - (Mouillé (e))
Wheal; hives - (Bouton, piqûre)
White - (Blanc)
White blood cell - (Globules blancs)
White coat - (Blouse de medecin, sarrau)
Whitlow; pale and sickly person - (Panaris)
Wide - (Large)
Widow - (Veuf/ Veuve)
Will - (Volonté)
Willis Circle - (Cercle de Willis)
Wilms tumor - (Tumeur de Wilms)
Wind - (Vent)
Window - (Fenêtre)
Window, therapeutic - (Éventail thérapeutique)
Wine - (Vin)
Woman - (Femme)
Womb - (Ventre)
Womb; uterus - (Matrice, utérus)

Work - (Travailler)
Work environment - (Environnement de travail)
Work injuries - (Accident de travail)
Working Conditions - (Conditions de travail)
Working hours - (Heure de consultation)
World Health Organization - (Organisation Mondiale de laSanté)
Worm - (Ver)
Worse - (Pire)
Worsen, to - (Empirer)
Wound; injury - (Blessure)
Wounded - (Blessé)
Wrinkles of the skin - (Rides de la peau)
Wrist - (Poignet)

~ X ~

Xanthelasma - (Xanthélasma)
Xanthem - (Xanthome)
Xanthema - (Xanthome)
Xanthomatosis - (Xanthomatose)
Xerophagia - (Xérophagie)
Xerophthalmia - (Xérophtalmie)
Xerostomia - (Xérostomie)
Xerostomia (dry mouth) - (Hyposalivation)

Xerotocia - (Accouchement á sec)
Xiphoid - (Xiphoïde)
Xiphoid apophysis - (Apophyse xiphoïde)
Xoderma - (Xérodermie)
X-rays - (Rayon X)

~ Y ~

Year - (An)
Yellow - (Jaune)
Yellow fever - (Fièvre jaune)
Yellowish - (Jaunâtre)

Yesterday - (Hier)
Yoga - (Yoga)
Yogurt - (Yogourt)
Young person - (Jeune)
Youth - (Jeunesse)

~ Z ~

Zero - (Zéro)
Zone - (Zona)
Zoonosis - (Zoonose)
Zoster - (Zona)
Zygote - (zygote)

Français - English

~ A ~

A jeun - (Fast (go without eating))
A jeun - (go without eating)
A l'intérieur, en dedans - (Inside)
Abactérien - (Abacterial)
Abattu - (Depressed)
abcès - (abscess)
Abcès périamygdalien - (Peritonsillar abscess)
Abdomen - (Abdomen)
Abdominal - (Abdominal)
Abdominocentèse - (Abdominocentesis)
Abdominogénital - (Abdominogenital)
Abduction - (Abduction)
Aberrant - (Aberrant)
Aberration - (Aberration)
Ablactation - (Ablaction)
Ablation - (Ablation)
Ablation de la rétine - (Retinal ablation)
Abondant - (Abundant)
Abondant - (plentiful)
Abondant - (Profuse)
Abortif (tive - (Abortifacient)
Abrasion - (Abrasion)
Abriter - (Cover)
Abriter - (keep warm)
Abrupt (e - (Abrupt)
Abruption du placenta - (Placenta abruptia)
Absence - (Absence)
Absence de réflexe - (Areflexia)
Absorption - (Absorption)
Abstème - (Abstemious)
Abstinence - (Abstinence)
Abus - (Abuse)
Abus de drogues - (Drug abuse)
Abus de médicaments - (Medication abuse)
Abus sexuel - (Sexual abuse)
Abus sur des enfants - (Child abuse)
Académique - (Academic)
acaricide - (acaricide)

Acarus - (mite)
Acarus - (Parasite)
Accablement - (fatigued)
Accablement -
(Overwhelmed)
Accélérer la guérison -
(Healing, to speed the
process of)
Accès - (Access)
Accident - (Accident)
Accident - (Crash)
Accident de la route -
(Transit accidents)
Accident de travail - (Work
injuries)
Accident domestiques -
(Accidents at home)
Accidenté(e - (Injured
person)
Accidenter - (Accident;
crash)
Accommodation -
(Accommodation)
Accommoder -
(Accommodate, to; adjust,
to)
Accompagnateur -
(Companion)
Accomplissement -
(Accomplishment)
Accord - (Agreement)
Accorder - (Agree, to)
Accouchement - (birth)

Accouchement - (Delivery)
Accouchement à domicile -
(Birth, home)
Accouchement á sec - (dry
birth)
Accouchement á sec -
(Xerotocia)
Accoucher - (Give birth, to)
Accroupi - (Squatting)
Accumulation -
(Accumulation)
Acétabule - (Acetabulum)
Acétabule - (hip socket)
Acétone - (Acetone)
Acétonurie - (Acetonuria)
Acetylcholine -
(Acetylcholine)
Acide - (Acid)
Acide ascorbique - (Ascorbic
acid)
Acide carbonique -
(Carbonic acid)
Acide chlorhydrique -
(Chlorhydric acid)
Acide désoxirhydrique -
(Deoxyribonucleic acid)
Acide folique - (Folic acid)
Acide nucléique - (Nucleic
acid)
Acide salicylique - (Salicylic
acid)
Acide urique - (Uric acid)
Acidité - (Acidity)

Acidité - (heartburn)
Acidité - (sour stomach)
Acidité gastrique - (Gastric acid)
Acidose - (Acidemia)
Acidose - (Acidosis)
Acidose diabétique - (Diabetic acidosis)
Acinus - (Acinus)
Acné - (Acne)
Acouphène - (Tinnitus)
Acouphène - (Tinnitus)
Acrocyanose - (Acrocyanosis)
Acromégalie - (Acromegaly)
Acromion - (Acromion)
Acte - (Certificate)
Acte - (official document)
ACTH - (ACTH)
Actif(ve - (Active)
Activeur - (Activator)
Activir - (Acyclovir)
activir - (antiviral)
Activité - (Activity)
Acuité - (Acuity)
Acuité visuelle - (Visual acuity)
Acupuncture - (Acupuncture)
Adaptation - (Adaptation)
Adducteur - (Adductor)
Adduction - (Adduction)

Adénite - (Adenitis)
Adénite - (inflamed gland)
Adénocarcinome - (Adenocarcinoma)
Adénoïde - (Adenoid)
Adénoïdectomie - (Adenoidectomy)
Adénoïdien - (Adenoid)
Adénoïdite - (Adenoiditis)
Adénome - (Adenoma)
Adénopathie - (Adenopathy)
Adéquat(e - (Adequate)
Adhérence - (Adhesion)
Adipose - (adipose)
Adipose - (Fatty)
Administration - (Administration)
Administration des services de santé - (Health services administration)
Administration publique - (Public administration)
Administration sanitaire - (Health administration)
Administrer un médicament - (Medication, to give a)
Admission - (Admission)
Admission de patients - (Admission of patients)
Adolescence - (Adolescence)
Adolescent - (Adolescent)

Adrénaline - (Adrenaline)
Adrénergique - (Adrenal)
Adrénocorticotropine -
(Adrenocorticotropin)
Adulte - (Adult)
Adverse, contraire -
(Adverse)
Aérobie - (Aerobe)
Aérogastrie - (Aerogastria)
Aérophagie - (Aerophagia)
Aérosol - (Aerosol)
Aérosol - (spray)
Affamé (e - (Starving)
Affecté au cœur - (Affected
by a heart condition)
Affectés par le SIDA -
(Affected by AIDS)
Affection - (Affection)
Affection - (condition)
Affection - (disease)
Afférent - (Afferent)
Affinité - (Affinity)
Affliction - (Affliction)
Affliction - (grief)
Agalactie - (Agalorrhea)
Age - (Age)
Agénésie - (Agenesis)
Agent - (Agent)
Agent causal - (Causal
agent)
Agent infectieux -
(Infectious agent)
Agent tératogène -

(Teratogenic agent)
Agglutination -
(Agglutination)
Agglutinogène -
(Agglutinogen)
Agir - (Act, to)
Agitation - (agitation)
Agitation - (Excitement)
Agité(e - (Anxious)
Agité(e - (uneasy)
Agiter - (Agitate, to)
Agiter - (shake, to)
Agonie - (anguish)
Agonie - (Suffering)
Agrandissement -
(Enlargement)
Agranulocytose -
(Agranulocytosis)
Agressif (ve - (Aggressive)
Aide - (Assistant)
Aide alimentaire - (food aid)
Aide alimentaire - (Relief,
food)
Aigre - (Sour)
Aiguille - (Needle)
Aine - (Groin)
Air - (Air)
Aisselle - (Armpit)
aisselle - (axilla)
Ajuster - (Adjust, to)
Alarmant, inquiétant -
(Alarming)
Alarme - (Alarm)

Albinos - (Albino)
Albumine - (Albumin)
Albuminurie - (Albuminuria)
Alcaloïde - (Alkaloid)
Alcalose - (Alkalosis)
Alcool - (Alcohol)
Alcoolémie - (alcoholemy)
Alcoolémie - (Blood alcohol)
Alcoolique - (Alcoholic)
Alcoolisme - (Alcoholism)
Aldostérone - (Aldosterone)
Alerte - (Alert)
Algie - (Algia)
Algorithme - (Algorhithm)
Alimentaire - (Related to food)
Alimentation - (Diet)
Alimentation supplémentaire - (Dietary supplement)
Alimentation thérapeutique - (Therapeutic diet)
Alimenter - (Feed, to)
Aliments - (Food)
Allaitement - (Lactation)
Allaitement maternel - (Breastfeeding)
Allaiter - (Breastfeed)
Allaiter, téter - (Lactate, to)
Allantoïdes - (Allantois)
Allergène - (Allergen)
Allergie - (Allergy)
Allergique - (Allergic)

Allergologiste - (Allergist)
Alopécie - (Alopecia)
Alpha fœto- protéine - (Alpha fetoprotein)
Altérer - (Alter)
Altérer - (modify)
Alternative - (Alternative)
Alvéolaire - (Alveolar)
Alvéole - (Alveolus)
Alvéolite - (Alveolitis)
Amaigrissement - (Slimming; weight loss)
Amalgame - (Amalgam)
Amaurose - (Amaurosis)
Amblyopie - (Amblyopia)
Ambulance - (Ambulance)
Ambulatoire, dispensaire - (Ambulatory)
Amélioration - (Improvement)
Aménorrhée - (Amenorreha)
Amer(ère - (Bitter)
Amétropie - (Ametropia)
Amibe - (Ameba)
Amibiase - (Amebiasis)
Amidon - (Starch)
Aminoacides - (Amino acids)
Aminoacides essentiels - (Amino acids, Essential)
Amnésie - (Amnesia)
Amnésique - (Amnesiac)
Amniocentèse -

(Amniocentesis)
Amnios - (Amnios)
Amniotique - (Amniotic)
Amollissement - (Softening)
Amphétamine -
(Amphetamine)
Ampicilline - (Ampicilin)
Ampoule - (Vial; blister)
Amputation - (Amputation)
Amputer - (Amputate)
Amygdale - (Tonsillar)
Amygdalectomie -
(Tonsillectomy)
Amygdalectomie -
(Tonsillectomy)
Amygdales - (Tonsils)
Amygdalite - (Tonsilitis)
Amygdalite - (Tonsillitis)
Amylase - (Amylase)
An - (Year)
Anabolisant - (Anabolic)
Anaérobie - (Anaerobic)
Anaérobiose -
(Anaerobiosis)
Anal - (Anal)
Analgésie - (Analgesia)
Analgésique - (Analgesic)
Analogue - (Analogic)
Analphabète - (Illiterate)
Analyse - (Analysis)
Analyse des aliments -
(Nutritional analysis)
Analyse du sang - (Blood
analysis)
Analyse sanguin - (Blood
analysis)
Analyser - (Analyze)
Anaphylactique -
(Anaphylactic)
Anaphylaxie - (Anaphylaxis)
Anasarque - (Anasarca)
Anastomose -
(Anastomosis)
Anatomie - (Anatomy)
Anatomique - (Anatomic)
Androgène - (Androgenous)
Androgène - (Androgenous)
Anémie - (Anemia)
anémie - (anaemia)
Anémie falciforme -
(Anemia, Sickle cell)
Anémie falciforme - (Sickle
cell anemia)
Anémique, anémié -
(Anemic)
Anencéphale -
(Anencephaly)
Anergie - (Anergy)
Anesthésie - (Anesthesia)
Anesthésier - (Anesthetize)
Anesthésique - (Anesthetic)
anesthésique - (anaesthetic
)
anesthésique local - (local
anaesthetic)
Anesthésiste -

(Anesthesiologist)
Anévrisme - (Aneurysm)
Angéite - (Angitis)
Angine - (Angina)
Angine de poitrine - (Angina pectoris)
Angine instable - (Angina, unstable)
Angio oedème - (Angioedema)
Angiographie - (Angiography)
Angiome - (Angioma)
Angioplastie - (Angioplasty)
Angoisse - (Anxiety)
Animal - (Animal)
Aniscorie - (Anisocoria)
Ankylose - (Ankylosis)
Ankylosé - (Ankylosed)
Ankyloser - (Stiffen)
Ankylostome - (Hookworm)
Anniversaire - (Birthday)
Annulaire - (Ring finger)
Annulaire - (Ring finger)
Anomalie congénitale - (Congenital anomaly)
Anorexie - (Anorexia)
Anormal - (Abnormal)
Anormal - (Abnormal)
Anormalité - (Abnormality)
Anosmie - (Anosmia)
Anovulatoire - (Anovulatory)

Anoxie - (Anoxia)
Antagonisme - (Antagonism)
Ante cubital - (Antecubital)
Antérieur - (Anterior)
Anthrax - (Anthrax)
Anti arythmique - (Antiarrhythmic)
Anti convulsif (ve - (Anticonvulsive)
Anti dépressif - (Antidepressant)
Anti diarrhéique - (Anti-diarrhea)
Anti hypertenseur (se - (Antihypertensive)
Anti inflammatoire - (Anti-inflamatory)
Antiacide - (Antacid)
Antiagrégant plaquettaire - (Antiplatelet)
Antiallergique - (Anti-allergic)
Antiasthmatique - (Anti-asthmatic)
Antibiogramme - (Antibiogram)
Antibiotique - (Antibiotic)
antibiotique - (antibiotic)
Anticancéreux - (Anti-cancer)
Anticoagulant -

(Anticoagulant)
Anticorps - (Antibody)
anticorps - (antibody)
Antidote - (Antidote)
Antiémétique - (Antiemetic)
Antifongique - (Antifungal)
Antigène - (Antigen)
antigène - (antigen)
Antigrippal - (Anti-flu)
Antihelminthique -
(Anthelmintic)
Antihistaminique -
(Antihistamine)
Antihygiénique -
(Unhygienic)
Anti-inflammatoire non
stéroïdien - (Non-steroidal
anti-inflammatories;
NSAIDs)
Antimicrobien -
(Antibacterial)
Antimigraineux -
(Antimigrainous)
Antinéoplasique -
(Antineoplastic)
Antiparasitaire -
(Antiparasitic)
Antipoliomyélitique - (Anti-
polio)
Antipyrétique - (Antipyretic)
Antirétroviral -
(Antiretroviral)
Antisepsie - (Antisepsis)

Antiseptique - (Antiseptic)
antiseptique - (antiseptic)
antisérum - (antiserum)
Antispasmodique -
(Antispasmodic)
Antitoxine - (Antitoxin)
Antituberculeux -
(Antituberculous)
Antivariolique - (Antivariolic)
Antiviral - (Antiviral)
Antivirus - (Antiviral)
Antre, cavité organique -
(Cavity)
Anurie - (Anuria)
Anus - (Anus)
anus - (anus)
Anxiété - (Anxiety)
Anxieux - (Anxious)
Anxiolytique - (Sedative)
Aorte - (Aorta)
Aortique - (Aortic)
Apaiser, Calmer - (Sedate,
to)
Apaiser, pallier - (Palliate)
Aphasie - (Aphasia)
Aphone - (Aphonic)
Aphonie - (Aphonia; loss of
voice)
Aphrodisiaque -
(Aphrodisiac)
Aphte - (Aphtha; small
ulcer)
Apicectomie - (Apicectomy)

Aplasie - (Aplasia)
Apnée - (Apnea)
Aponévrose - (Aponeurosis)
Apophyse - (Apophysis)
Apophyse xiphoïde -
(Xiphoid apophysis)
Apoplexie - (Apoplexy)
Apoplexie - (Apoplexy)
Apoplexie embolique -
(Apoplexy, embolic)
Apoplexie hémorragique -
(Apoplexy, hemorrhagic)
Appareil acoustique -
(Hearing aid; auditory
apparatus)
Appareil digestif - (Digestive
system)
Appareil respiratoire -
(Respiratory system)
Apparence - (Appearance)
Appendice - (Appendix)
Appendicite - (Appendicitis)
Appétit - (Appetite)
Applicateur - (Applicator)
Application topique -
(Topical application)
Appliquer - (Apply)
Approprié(e - (Appropriate)
Approvisionnement
d'aliments - (Food supply)
Approvisionnement d'eau -
(Water supply)

Approvisionner, ravitailler -
(Supply, to)
Approximativement -
(Approximately)
Appui - (Help; aid;
assistance)
Aqueux(se - (Watery;
aqueous)
Arbovirus - (Arbovirus)
Ardeur - (Burning sensation)
Aréole - (Areola)
Arrêt - (Arrest (as in cardiac
or respiratory arrest))
Arrêt cardiaque - (Arrest,
cardiac)
Arrêt respiratoire - (Arrest,
respiratory)
Arrêter - (Stop, to)
Arrière grand-père
/Arrièregrand-mère - (Great
Grandfather / Great
Grandmother)
Arrière petit fils /Arrière
petitefille - (Great Grandson
/ Great Grandmother)
Arriver - (Happen, to)
Artère - (Artery)
artère - (artery)
Artères coronaires -
(Coronary arteries)
Artériosclérose -
(Arteriosclerosis)

Arthralgie - (Arthralgia)
Arthrite - (Arthritis)
arthrite - (arthritis)
Arthritique - (Arthritic)
Arthroscopie - (Arthroscopy)
Arthrose - (Arthrosis)
Articulation - (Joint)
Articulation - (Joint)
Artificiel - (Artificial)
Arythmie - (Arrhythmia)
Arythmie supra ventriculaire - (Supraventricular arrhythmia)
Arythmie ventriculaire - (Ventricular arrhythmia)
Ascaridiase - (Ascariasis)
Ascaridiose - (Ascariasis)
ascaris - (roundworms)
Ascendance - (Ascendance)
Ascite - (Ascites)
Asepsie - (Asepsis)
Aseptique - (Aseptic)
Asile des aliénés - (Asylum; psychiatric hospital)
Aspiration - (Aspiration)
Aspirer - (Aspirate)
Aspirine - (Aspirin)
Assez - (Enough)
Assis(se - (Seated; sitting (adj))
Assistance - (Assistance)
Assistance dentaire - (Dental assistance)
Assistance médicale - (Medical assistance)
Assistance publique - (Public assistance)
Assistant - (Attendent; assistant)
Assister - (Assist; attend)
Association - (Association)
Asthénie - (Asthenia)
Asthénie, adynamie - (Adynamia)
Asthmatique - (Asthmatic)
Asthme - (Asthma)
Astigmatisme - (Astigmatism)
Astringent - (Astringent)
Asymétrique - (Asymmetrical)
Asymptomatique - (Asymptomatic)
Asystolie - (Heart failure)
Ataxie - (Ataxia)
Atélectasie - (Atelactasis)
Athérome - (Atheroma)
Athétose - (Athetosis)
Atomiseur - (Atomizer)
Atrésie - (Atresia)
Atrioventriculaire - (Atrioventricular)
Atrophie - (Atrophy)
Atropine - (Atropine)
Atteint de syphilis - (Syphilitic)

Atteint du mal de mer - (Sea-sick, dizzy)
Atteinte d'insomnie - (Insomniac)
Attention - (Care)
Attrait - (Collection; reception)
Attraper une grippe - (Cold, to catch a)
Auditif - (Auditory)
Audition - (Hearing)
Aujourd'hui - (Today)
Aura - (Aura)
Auriculaire - (Auricular)
Auriculaire - (Little finger; pinky)
Auriculaire, petit doigt - (Pinkie; little finger)
Auscultation - (Auscultation)
Auscultation médicale - (Medical examination)
Auscultation, examen - (Examination; recognition)
Ausculter - (Auscultate)
Auto soins, se soigner soimême - (Self-Care)
Auto-immune - (Auto-immune)
Automatisme - (Automatism)
Automédication - (Self-Medication)

Autonome - (Autonomous)
Autopsie - (Autopsy)
Autoriser la sortie de l'hôpital - (Release from hospital)
Autosome - (Autosomatic)
Autre - (Other)
Auxiliaire, aide infirmière - (Nurse's Assistant)
Avaler - (Swallow)
Avance, progrès - (Advance)
Avant bras - (Forearm)
Avant la fin - (Preterm)
Aveugle - (Blind)
Avitaminose - (Avitaminosis)
Avoir un accident - (Accident, to have an)
Avoir une bonne vue - (Good visibility, to have)
Avoir une crise cardiaque - (Attack, Heart, to have a)
Avorté(e - (Aborted)
Avortement - (Abortion; miscarriage)
Avorter - (Abort; miscarry, to)
Axone - (Axon)
Azoospermie - (Azoospermia)
Azotémie - (Azotemia)

~ B ~

Bacillus, bactérie - (Bacillus)
Bactericide, germicide - (Bactericidal)
Bactérie - (Bacteria)
Bactérie fécale coliforme - (Bacteria, fecal coliform)
Bactériémie - (Bacteremia)
Bactériémique - (Bacteremic)
Bactérien - (Bacterial)
bactéries - (bacteria)
Bactériologiste - (Bacteriologist)
Bactérionurie - (Bacteriuria)
Bactériostatique - (Bacteriostatic)
Badigeonnage - (Strokes, brush)
Baigner - (Bathe, to)
Bain - (Bath)
Balance - (Balance)
Balance - (Scale (for weighing) [as noun]; weighs [verb])
Balançoire - (Chair (armchair))
Balanite - (Balanitis)
Balanopostite - (Balanoposthitis)
Bandage - (Bandage)

Bandage - (Bandage)
Bande réactive - (Dipstick)
Banque de sang - (Blood supply)
Banque de sang - (Bloodbank)
Barbiturique - (Barbiturate)
Barorécepteur - (Baroreceptor)
Barrière - (Barrier)
Bas(se - (Low)
Basal - (Basal)
Base - (Base)
Base de données - (Database)
Basophile - (Basophilic)
Bassin, pelvis - (Pelvis)
Battement - (Beat (as in heart beat))
Battement cardiaque rythmique - (Beat, rythmic cardiac)
Beau père/ Belle mère - (Father-in-Law)
Bébé - (Baby)
Bebé, Nouveau-né - (Baby)
Bec - (Mouthpiece; snack (reg))
Bégayer - (Suttering; stammering)
Bègue - (Stutterer)
Belladone - (Belladonna)
Bénéfice - (Benefit)

Bénéfice - (Profit)
Bénévole - (Volunteer)
Bénin - (Benign)
Benzocaïne - (Benzocaine)
Béquilles - (Crutches)
Berceau - (Cradle)
Béribéri - (Beriberi)
berseem - (berseem)
Beurre - (Butter)
Biberon - (Baby bottle)
Bibliographie -
(Bibliography)
Bibliothèque - (Library)
Biceps - (Biceps)
Bicuspid - (Bicuspid)
Bien - (Good)
Bien-être - (Wellbeing)
Bien-être social - (Social
wellbeing)
Bienvenu(e - (Welcome)
Bigamie - (Bigamy)
Bilan de santé, check-up -
(Medical check-up)
Bilatéral (e - (Bilateral)
Bile - (Bile)
Biliaire - (Biliary)
Biliaire - (Vesical)
Bilirubine - (Bilirubin)
Bilirubinémie -
(Bilirubinemia)
Bimanuel - (Bimanual)
Biochimie - (Biochemistry)

Biocompatibilité -
(Biocompatible)
Biodégradation -
(Biodegradable)
Biodisponibilité -
(Bioavailability)
Bioéquivalent -
(Bioequivalent)
Biologie - (Biology)
Biométrie hématique -
(Blood Biometric)
Biopsie - (Biopsy)
Biostatistique - (Biostatistic)
Biosynthèse - (Biosyntesis)
Biotine - (Biotin)
Biotype - (Biotype)
Bipède - (Biped)
Bisexuel - (Bisexual)
Bistouri - (Scapel)
Bizarre - (Rare)
Bizarre, rare - (Strange;
foreign)
Blanc - (White)
Blennorragie - (Gonorrhea)
Blépharite - (Blepharitis)
Blépharo-conjonctivite -
(Blepharo-conjuntivitis)
Blépharoplégie -
(Blepharoplegia)
Blépharoptose -
(Blepharoptosis)
Blépharospame -

(Blepharospasm)
Blessé - (Wounded)
Blessé par balle - (Gunshot wound)
Blesser, faire mal - (Damage, to; injure)
Blessure - (Wound; injury)
Blessure par arme blanche - (Stab wound)
Bleu - (Blue)
Bleu - (Bruise; purple)
blister - (blister)
Blocus - (Blockade (as in anesthetic regional block))
Blouse de medecin, sarrau - (White coat)
blowfly - (blowfly)
Boire - (Drink, to)
Boire, prendre, prélever - (Take)
Boiter, clocher - (Limp)
Boiteux - (Lame)
boiteux - (lame)
Bomber - (Bulge; make bulge, to)
Bon diagnostic - (Correct diagnosis)
Bon marché, pas cher - (Cheap)
Bon/Bonne - (Good)
Bonne practique - (Good practice)
Borgne - (One-eyed)

Bosse - (Hump)
Bosse - (Lump)
Botulisme - (Botulism)
Bouche - (Mouth)
Bouger - (Move, to)
Bouillie - (Pap (soft food))
Bouillir - (Boil, to)
Bouillon - (Soup; broth)
Bouillotte - (Hot water bottle)
Bourdonnement - (Buzzing)
Bourdonnement des oreilles - (Ears, ringing in the)
Bouteille - (Bottle)
Bouton - (Pimple; spot)
Bouton de chaleur - (Rash)
Bouton, piqûre - (Wheal; hives)
Bradycardie - (Bradycardia)
Bradypnée - (Bradypnea)
Brancard - (Stretcher)
Branche - (Branch)
Bras - (Arm)
Brisé(e), cassé(e - (Broken)
bronche - (bronchus)
Bronchectasie - (Bronchiectasis)
Bronchite - (Bronchiolitis)
Broncho pneumonie - (Bronchopneumonia)
Broncho-aspiration - (Bronchial aspiration)
Bronchodilatateur -

(Bronchodilator)
Bronchopulmonaire - (Bronchopulmonary)
Bronchorrhée - (Bronchorrhea)
Bronchotomie - (Bronchiotomy)
Broncoscopie - (Bronchoscope)
Brosse - (Brush)
Brosse à dents - (Toothbrush)
Brucellose - (Brucellosis)
Bruit - (Noise)
Bruit cardiaque - (Heart noise)
Brûlé (e - (Burned)
Brûlure d'estomac - (Heartburn)
Brûlures - (Burns)
Bruxomanie - (Bruxism)
Buccal - (Buccal)
Burdizzo outil pour la castration des animaux - (burdizzo)
Bursite - (Bursitis)
Buste - (Chest)
But - (Goal; aim)

~ C ~

Caca, selles, fèces - (Feces; fecal matter; shit)
Caché (e - (Hidden)
Cacher - (Hide, to)
Cachexie - (Cachexia)
Cadavre - (Cadaver)
Caecum - (Cecum)
caecum - (caecum)
Cage thoracique - (Thoracic cage)
Cagneux - (Bowlegged)
caillette - (abomasum)
caillot - (clot)
Caillot de sang - (Blood clot)
Calamine - (Calamine)
Calcémie - (Calcemia)
Calcification - (Calcification)
Calcium - (Calcium)
Calcul rénal - (Kidney stone)
Calcul, pierre - (Stone)
Callosité - (Corpus callosum)
Calmant - (Calming; that which calms)
Calmer - (Calm, to)
Calorie - (Calorie)
Calvitie - (Baldness)
Camarade, collègue - (Partner)
Campagne de promotion desanté - (Health promotion campaign)

Campagne de vaccination - (Vaccination campaign)
Canal - (Canal)
Canal déférent - (Deferent duct)
Canaliser - (Channel, to)
Cancer - (Cancer)
Cancer disséminé - (Metastisized cancer)
Cancer terminal - (Terminal cancer)
Cancéreux - (Cancerous)
Cancérigène - (Carcinogen)
Candida - (Candida)
Candidiase - (Candidiasis)
Canin - (Canine tooth)
Canine - (Canine tooth)
Canne, bâton - (Cane)
Canule - (Cannula)
Capable - (Capable)
Capacité - (Capacity)
Capacité vitale - (Vital capacity)
Capsule - (Capsule)
Capsule articulaire - (Articular capsule)
Caractère - (Character)
Caractère de ce qui est rugueux - (Roughness)
Carbohydrate - (Carbohydrate)
Carcinogène - (Carcinogen)
Carcinome - (Carcinoma)

Carcinome du chorion - (Choriocarcinoma)
Cardia - (Cardiac)
Cardialgie - (Cardialgia)
Cardiaque - (Cardiac)
Cardinal - (Cardinal)
Cardiogramme - (Cardiogram)
Cardiographie - (Cardiograph)
Cardiologie - (Cardiology)
Cardiologue - (Cardiologist)
Cardiomégalie - (Cardiomegaly)
Cardiomégalie - (Cardiomegaly)
Cardiomyopathie - (Cardiomyopathy)
Cardio-pulmonaire - (Cardiopulmonary)
Cardiotonique - (Cardiotonic)
Cardiovasculaire - (Cardiovascular)
Cardioversion - (Cardioverson)
Carence - (Lack of; deficiency)
Carie dentaire - (Cavities (dental))
Carotène - (Carotene)
Carotide - (Carotid)
Carotinémie - (Carotenemia)

Carpe - (Carpus)
Cartilage - (Cartilage)
Caryotype - (Karyotype)
Cas - (Case)
Cas index - (Case index)
Cassé (e - (Broken)
Casser, briser - (Break, to)
Casser, se casser - (Break, to)
Cassure - (Fracture; tear; breakage)
Catabolisme - (Catabolism)
Catalepsie - (Catalepsy)
Cataliser - (Catalyze, to)
Cataplasme - (Cataplasm)
cataplasme - (poultice)
Cataracte - (Cataract)
Catarrhal - (Catarrhal)
Catastrophe naturelle - (Natural catasrophe)
Catécholamine - (Catecholamine)
Cathéter - (Catheter)
Caudal - (Caudal; volume of flow)
Causal - (Causal)
Cause - (Cause)
cautériser - (cauterise)
Cave - (Cave)
Caverne - (Cavern)
Caverne pulmonaire - (Lung cavity)

Cavité - (Cavity)
Cavité orale - (Oral cavity)
Cecité - (Blindness)
Cellule - (Cell)
Cellullite - (Cellulitis)
Centigrade - (Centigrade)
Centimètre - (Centimeter)
Central - (Central)
Centre - (Center)
Centre de planification familiale - (Family Planning Center)
Centre de rééducation - (Rehabilitation center)
Centre de santé - (Health Center)
Centre de santé publique - (Public health center)
Céphalée - (Cephalia)
Céphalexine - (Cephalexin)
Céphalique - (Cephalic)
Céphalosporine - (Cephalosporin)
Cerclage - (Cerclage)
Cercle - (Circle)
Cercle de Willis - (Willis Circle)
Cercueil - (Casket)
Cérébro-spinal - (Cerebrospinal)
Cérébrovasculaire - (Cerebrovascular)

Certificat - (Certificate)
Certificat de décès - (Death certificate)
Certificat de décès - (Death certificate)
Certificat de naissance, actede naissance - (Birth certificate)
Certificat de santé - (Health certificate)
Certificat médical - (Medical certificate)
Certifier une mort - (Certify a death, to)
Cérumen - (Earwax)
Cerveau - (Brain)
Cervelet - (Cerebellum)
Cervelet-spinal - (Cerebellospinal)
Cervical - (Cervical)
Cervical, relatif au cou - (Cervix)
Cervicite - (Cervicitis)
Césarienne - (Cesarean)
Cestoïde - (Tapeworm)
Cetoacidose - (Ketoacidosis)
Cetose - (Ketosis)
Chaise - (Chair)
Chalazion - (Chalazion)
Chaleur - (Heat)
Chambre - (Room)
Chambre de malade - (Patient room)

Chambre de soins - (Treatment room)
Champ visuel - (Visual field)
champignon - (fungus)
Champion qui pousse sur lesplantes - (Diplodia)
Chancre - (Chancre)
Change - (Change)
changer - (Alter)
changer - (modify)
Charbon - (Carbon)
Châtré - (Castrated)
Châtrer - (Castrate, to)
Chaud - (Hot)
Chéilite - (Cheilitis)
Cheilose - (Cheilosis)
Chéloïde - (Keloid)
Chemise - (Shirt)
Chercher - (Look for, to)
Cheveux - (Hair)
Cheville - (Ankle)
Cheville - (Malleolus)
Chicot - (Root (of a tooth))
Chimie - (Chemistry)
Chimio prophylaxie - (Chemoprophylaxis)
Chimiorécepteur - (Chemoreceptor)
Chimiothérapie - (Chemotherapy)
Chimiste - (Chemist)
Chiropraxie - (Chiropraxis; chiropractic)

Chirurgical (e - (Surgical)
Chirurgie - (Surgery)
Chirurgien - (Surgeon)
Chlamydia - (Chlamydia)
Chloasme - (Chloasma)
Chloroquine - (Chloroquine)
Chlorpromazine -
(Chlorpromazine)
choc - (accident)
choc - (Crash)
Choc anaphylactique -
(Anaphylactic shock)
Cholangite - (Cholangitis)
Cholecystectomie -
(Choleystectomy)
Cholecystite - (Cholecystitis)
Cholédoque - (Choledochus)
Cholélitiase - (Cholelithiasis)
Choléra - (Cholera)
Cholestase - (Cholestasis)
Cholestérol - (Cholesterol)
Cholinergique -
(Cholinergic)
Chorée - (Chorea)
Chorion - (Chorion; corium)
Chromatine - (Chromatine)
Chromosome -
(Chromosome)
Chromosome asexuel -
(Asexual chromosome)
Chromosome sexuel -
(Sexual chromosome)

Chronicité - (Chronicity)
Chronique - (Chronic)
Chute - (Fall)
Cicatrice - (Scar)
Cicatrisation - (Scar
formation)
Cicle menstrual - (Menstrual
cycle)
Ciclique - (Cyclical)
Cigarette - (Cigarette)
Cil - (Eyelash)
Ciller - (Ciliary)
Cinquième - (Fifth)
Circoncision - (Circumcision)
Circulation - (Circulation)
Cirrhose - (Cirrhosis)
Ciseaux - (Scissors)
Clair(e - (Clear; Okay)
Classe - (Classroom)
Classification -
(Classification)
Claudification intermittente
- (Claudication, intermittent)
Clavicule - (Clavicle)
Clignement des yeux -
(Blink)
Climat - (Climate)
Clinique - (Clinic)
Clinique - (Clinical)
Clitoris - (Clitoris)
Cloison - (Septum)
Cloison nasale, septum

nasal - (Septum)
Clonage - (Cloning)
Clone - (Clone)
CMV-cytomégalovirus -
(CMV; Cytomegalovirus)
Coagulation - (Coagulation)
Cocaïne - (Cocaine)
Coccyx - (Coccyx)
Coccyx - (Coccyx)
Codéine - (Codeine)
Coeliaque - (Celiac)
Cœur - (Heart)
Cohérent - (Coherent)
Coït - (Coitus)
col - (cervix)
Col de l'utérus - (Cervix)
Colectomie - (Colectomy)
Colique - (Colic)
coliques - (colic)
Colite - (Colitis)
Colite ulcéreuse - (Colitis,
ulcerative)
Collagénose - (Collagenosis)
Collapsus - (Collapse)
Collègue - (Colleague)
Collyre - (Collyrium)
Colon - (Colon)
Colonie - (Colony)
Coloniser - (Colonize)
Colonne vertébrale -
(Vertebral Column)
Coloration - (Coloration)
Colostomie - (Colostomy)

Colostrum - (Colostrum)
colostrum - (colostrum)
Colposcopie - (Colposcopy)
Coma - (Coma)
Comateux(euse -
(Comatose)
Combinaison -
(Combination)
Commencement, début -
(Begining)
Commotion - (Commotion)
Communauté -
(Community)
commune - (joint)
Compatible - (Compatible)
Compenser - (Compensate)
compenser - (compensate)
Complément -
(Complement)
Complication -
(Complication)
Compliqué - (Complicated)
Comportement - (Behavior)
Composition familiale -
(Family composition)
Comprendre -
(Comprehend)
Comprendre - (Understand)
Compresse - (Compress)
Comprimé - (Pill)
Comprimé - (Tablet)
Compte gouttes -
(Eyedropper)

Concentration - (Concentration)
Concept - (Concept)
Conception - (Conception)
Condition - (Condition)
Conditions de travail - (Working Conditions)
Conditions sociales - (Social conditions)
Condom - (Condom)
Conduction - (Conduction)
Conduit - (Conduit)
Conduit - (Duct)
Conduite, façon d'agir - (Actuation)
Condyle - (Condyle)
Condylome - (Condyloma)
Conférence - (Conference)
Confiance - (Confidence)
Confidentiel - (Confidential)
Confirmer - (Confirm, to)
Confus(e - (Confuse)
Confusion - (Confusion)
Congé de l'hôpital - (Hospital discharge)
Congénital (e - (Congenital)
Congestion - (Congestion)
Conjonctive - (Conjunctive)
Conjonctivite - (Conjunctivitis)
Connaissance - (Knowledge)
Connaître, savoir - (Know, to; meet, to)
Connection - (Connection)
Consanguinité - (Consanguinity)
Conscience - (Conscience)
Conscient - (Conscious)
Conscient - (Conscious)
Conseil - (Advice; counsel)
Conseil génétique - (Genetic Counseling)
Conseillé(e - (Advisable)
Conservation d'aliments - (Food Preservation)
Conserver - (Conserve)
Consommer - (Consume)
Constipation - (Constipation)
Constipation - (Constipation)
Constipé (e - (Constipated)
Constipé(e - (Constipated)
Constitution - (Constitution)
Consultation - (Doctor's appointment)
Consultation médicale à domicile - (Home medical visit; housecall)
Contact - (Contact)
Contagieux - (Contagious)
Contagion - (Contagion)
Contamination - (Contamination; pollution)

Contamination de l'eau
(del'air - (Water (Air)
contamination; pollution)
contaminer - (contaminate
)
Contenu - (Content)
Contraceptif -
(Contraceptive)
Contraception -
(Contraception)
Contraception -
(Contraceptive)
Contraception -
(Contraceptive)
Contracté(e - (Contracted)
Contractile - (Contractile)
Contraction - (Contraction)
Contraction muscles
abdominaux - (Abdominal
muscle contraction)
Contraction musculaire -
(Muscular contraction)
Contractions précoces -
(Premature contractions)
Contracture - (Contracture)
Contre - (Against)
Contre le mal de mer -
(Anti-motion sickness)
Contre-indication -
(Contraindication)
Contrôle d'insectes - (Insect
control)
Contrôle de fléaux - (Control

of plagues)
Contrôle de moustiques -
(Mosquito control)
Contrôle de rongeurs -
(Rodent control)
Contrôle des maladies
transmissibles - (Control of
transmitable diseases)
Contrôle des médicaments -
(Control of medicine; drugs)
Contrôle des médicaments
et narcotiques - (Control of
drugs and narcotics)
Contrôler - (Control)
Contusion - (Bruise)
Contusion - (Contusion)
Convalescence -
(Convalescence)
Convulsion - (Convulsion)
Convulsion fiévreuse -
(Febrile convulsion; seizure)
convulsions - (convulsions)
Coopérer - (Cooperate)
Coordonner - (Coordinate)
Coproculture -
(Coproculture)
Copule - (Copulation)
Coqueluche - (Pertussis;
whooping cough)
Coqueluche - (Pertussis;
whooping cough)
Cor, callosité - (Callus; corn)
Corde - (Cord)

Cordes vocales - (Vocal cords)
Cordon ombilical - (Umbilical cord)
cordon ombilical - (umbilical cord)
cordon spermatique - (spermatic cord)
Cornée - (Cornea)
cornée - (cornea)
Coronarien - (Coronary)
Corporel - (Corporal)
Corps - (Body)
Corps caverneux du pénis - (Cavernous body of the penis)
Corps de Barr - (Barr corpuscle)
Corps étranger - (Foreign body)
Corps jaune(corpus luteum - (Corpus luteum)
Corpuscule de Barr - (Barr corpuscle; Barr body)
Correct (e - (Correct)
Cortex - (Cortex)
Cortex cérébral - (Cerebral Cortex)
Corticostéroïdes - (Corticosteroids)
Corticotrophine - (Corticotropin)

Cortisol, hydro-cortisone - (Cortisol)
Côte - (Rib)
Coton - (Cotton)
Cou - (Neck)
Couche - (Diaper)
Coucher - (Lay down, to)
Coude - (Elbow)
Coup - (Blow)
Coupe - (Cut (noun))
Couper - (Cut (verb))
Courage - (Courage; state of mind)
Courbe - (Curve)
Couvercle, bouchon - (Cap)
Couverture - (Coverage)
Couveuse - (Incubator)
Couvrir - (Cover)
Couvrir - (Cover)
Coxalgie - (Coxalgia)
Coxofémoral - (Coxofemoral)
Crachat - (Sputum)
Crachat sanguinolente - (Bloody Sputum)
Crampe - (Cramp)
Crampes - (Cramps)
Crâne - (Cranium)
Crânien - (Cranial)
Créatinine - (Creatinine)
Crème - (Cream)
Crétinisme - (Cretinism,

hypothyroidism)
Cris - (Shout)
Crise - (Attack)
Crise - (Crisis)
Crise cardiaque - (Heart
attack)
Crise cardiaque - (Heart
attack)
Crise épileptique - (Epileptic
seizure)
Crise ischémique transitoire
- (Transient ischemic attack)
Crise nerveuse - (Nervous
breakdown)
Crise nerveuse - (Nervous
Breakdown)
Cristalisation -
(Crystalization)
Cristallin - (Lens)
Critère - (Criteria)
Croissance - (Growth)
Croix Rouge - (Red Cross)
Croûte - (Scab)
Cryochirurgie -
(Cryosurgery)
Cryptorchidie -
(Cryptorchidy)
Cubital - (Cubital)
Cubitus - (Ulna)
Cuisse - (Thigh)
Culture - (Testing; study)
culture - (crop)
Culture fécale, culture

deselles - (Fecal culture)
Cure - (Cure; priest (as one
curing souls))
Cure de repos - (Cure by
resting)
Curetage - (Curettage)
Curetage, avortement -
(Curettage)
Cyanose - (Cyanosis)
Cyanosé - (Cyanotic)
Cyclotimie - (Cyclothymia)
Cyphose - (Kyphosis)
Cystadenome -
(Cystadenoma)
Cystite - (Cystitis)
Cystoscopie - (Cystoscopy)
Cytologie - (Cytology)
Cytolyse - (Cytolysis)
Cytopénie - (Cytopenia)
Cytoplasme - (Cytoplasm)
Cytotoxique - (Cytotoxic)

~ B ~

Dacryocystite -
(Dacryocystitis)
Dactylite, inflammation
dudoigt - (Inflammation of
fingers)
Daltonien - (Colorblind)
Dangereux - (Dangerous)
Date - (Date)

Débôitement - (Dislocation)
Déboîter - (Dislocated)
Débridement -
(Debridement)
Début - (Beginning)
Décérébration -
(Decerebrate)
décharger - (discharge)
Déchet - (Waste)
Déchirement - (Tear)
Déciduale - (Decidual)
Décilitre - (Deciliter)
Décision - (Decision)
Décomposer - (Decompose)
Décomposition -
(Decomposition)
Décongestion -
(Decongestion)
Décongestionnant -
(Decongestant)
Décongestionner -
(Decongest, to)
Décontamination -
(Decontamination)
Décortication -
(Decortication)
Découragé, déprimé -
(Depressed)
Découvrir - (Discover)
Décroître - (Decrease)
Décubitus - (Lying)
Décubitus dorsal - (Supine;
lying face up)
Décubitus ventral - (Prone;
lying face down)
Dedans - (Inside)
Défaillance ventriculaire -
(Ventricular failure)
Défaillir, s'évanouir - (Faint;
pass out, to)
Défaut - (Defect; flaw)
Défaut de naissance - (Birth
defect)
Défécation - (Defecation;
bowel movement)
Défense - (Defense)
Déféquer - (Defecate, to)
Défibrillateur -
(Defibrillator)
Défibrillation -
(Defibrillation)
Déficience - (Deficiency)
Déficience nutritionnelle -
(Nutritional deficiency)
Déficience vitaminique -
(Vitamin deficiency)
Déficit - (Deficit)
Défloration - (Defloration)
Déformation -
(Deformation)
Dégénératif (ve -
(Degenerative)
Dégénérescence -
(Degeneration)

Dégénérescence maculaire - (Macular degeneration)
Déglutition - (Swallowing)
Dégoût - (Disgust; nausea)
Dégradation - (Degradation)
Degré - (Degree)
Déhiscence - (Dehiscence)
Dehors - (Outside)
Dehors, hors - (Outside of; out)
Déjeuner, dîner, lunch - (Lunch)
Délire - (Delirium)
Deltoïdes - (Deltoids)
Demain - (Tomorrow)
Démangeaison, picotement,prurit - (Itching, pruritus)
Démangeaison. picotement - (Itching)
Démence - (Dementia)
Démographie - (Demography)
Démonstration - (Demonstration; sign)
Démyélinisation - (Demyelination)
Dendrite - (Dendrite)
Dengue - (Dengue)
Dénomination - (Denomination)
Dent - (Tooth)
Dent de lait - (Baby teeth)

Dentifrice - (Toothpaste)
Dentiste - (Dentist)
Dentiste, stomatologue - (Stomatologist; dentist)
Dentition - (Dentition)
Dentition - (Denture)
Dentition définitive - (Fixed denture)
Dentition partielle - (Partial denture)
Dents permanentes - (Permanent teeth)
Déontologie - (Deontology)
Département - (Department)
Département des urgences - (Emergency department)
Dépendance - (Addiction)
Dépendance - (Dependency)
Dépendance du médicament - (Medicine dependence)
Dépendant - (Dependent)
Dépense - (Expense)
Dépersonnalisation - (Depersonalization)
Dépister - (Scan; tracking)
Déplacement - (Displacement)
Déplétion - (Depletion)
Dépotoir, dépôt - (Warehouse)
Dépression nerveuse -

(Nervous breakdown)
Dérivé(e - (Derived)
Dérivés du sang - (Blood products)
Dermatite - (Dermatitis)
Dermatite herpétiforme - (Herpetiforme dermatitis)
Dermatite irritante - (Skin irritation)
Dermatite séborique - (Seborrheic dermatitis)
Dermatologie - (Dermatology)
Dermatologique - (Dermatological)
Dermatologue - (Dermatologist)
Dermatomycose - (Dermatomycoses)
Dermatose - (Dermatosis)
Dermo candidiase - (Candidiasis of the skin)
Dernier (ère - (Last)
Derrière - (Behind)
Désajustement - (Dislocation)
Désarticuler - (Disarticulate)
Désastres - (Disasters)
Descendance - (Descendence)
Descendre - (Lower, to)
Désensibilisation -

(Desensitize)
Déséquilibre électrolytique - (Electrolytic imbalance)
Déshabiller, dénuder - (Remove all clothing; undress, to)
Déshydratation - (Dehydration)
déshydratation - (dehydration)
Déshydraté - (Dehydrated)
Désinfectant - (Disinfectant)
Désinfecter - (Disinfect, to)
Désinfection - (Disinfection)
Desinhibation - (Uninhibited)
Désintoxication - (Detoxification)
Désorienté - (Disoriented)
Desquamation - (Desquamation)
Dessous - (Underneath)
Détecter - (Detect, to)
Détection - (Detection)
Détendu (e - (Lax)
Détériorer - (Deteriorate)
Deux fois par jour - (B.I.D.; twice a day)
Deux fois par jour - (Twice a day)
Devant - (In front of)
Développement -

(Development)
Développement
d'anticorpsdétectables -
(Seroconversion)
Développement de l'enfant -
(Infantile development)
Développement fœtal -
(Fetal development)
Développer - (Develop)
Devenir rouge -
(Reddening)
Devenir virile - (Virilization;
masculinization)
Dévêtir - (Undress oneself)
Dexaméthasone -
(Dexamethasone)
Dextrocardie -
(Dextrocardia)
Dextrose - (Dextrose)
Diabète - (Diabetes)
Diabète mellitus - (Diabetes
Mellitus)
Diabétique - (Diabetic)
Diagnostic - (Diagnostic)
Diagnostic confirmé -
(Confirmed diagnosis)
Diagnostic prénatal -
(Prenatal diagnosis)
Diagnostiquer - (Diagnose)
Diaphorèse - (Diaphoresis,
sweat)
Diaphragme - (Diaphragm)
Diaphyse - (Diaphysis, shaft

of a bone)
Diarrhée - (Diarrhea)
diarrhée - (diarrhoea)
Diastole - (Diastole)
Diastolique - (Diastolic)
Diathèse - (Diathesis)
Dichotomie - (Dichotomy)
Dictionnaire - (Dictionary)
Dictionnaire de poche -
(Pocket dictionary)
Diencéphale -
(Diencephalon)
Diète - (Diet)
Différenciation -
(Differentiation)
Différer - (Defer)
Diffuse - (Diffuse; unclear)
Diffuser, reprendre -
(Diffuse, to; spread out, to)
Digérer - (Digest)
Digestif (ive - (Digestive)
Digestion - (Digestion)
digestion - (digestion)
Digital - (Digital)
Digitalisation -
(Digitalization)
Digitoxine - (Digitoxin)
Dilatation - (Dilatation)
Dilater - (Expand; dilate)
Dilution - (Dilution)
Diminuer - (Diminish;
reduce)
Diminution, baisse -

(Decrease)
Diphtérie - (Diphtheria)
Diplocoque - (Diplococcus)
Diplôme - (Title; degree)
Diplôme après licence -
(Post-doctorate; graduate
school (varies))
Diplôme de médecine -
(Medical Diploma)
Diplophonie - (Diplophonia)
Diplopie - (Diplopia)
Dipsomanie - (Dipsomania)
Direct - (Direct)
Discoïde - (Discoid)
Discussion - (Discussion)
dislocation - (dislocation)
Dispensaire - (Dispensary)
Dispersion - (Dispersion)
Disponibilité - (Availability)
Dispositif - (Device)
Disposition - (Disposition)
Disséminé(e -
(Disseminated)
Dissociation - (Dissociation)
Dissolution - (Dissolution)
Dissolvant - (Solvent)
Distal - (Distal)
Distension - (Distention)
Distribuer, partager -
(Distribute, to; share, to)
Distribution - (Distribution)
Diurèse - (Diuresis)

Diurétique - (Diuretic)
Diverticule - (Diverticulum)
Diverticulite - (Diverticulitis)
Diverticulose -
(Diverticulosis)
Dixième - (Tenth)
Docteur - (Doctor)
Docteure - (Doctor
(female))
Documents - (Documents)
Doigt - (Finger)
Doigts en griffes - (Claw
hand)
Domicile - (Residence,
address)
Dominant - (Dominant)
Domination, Contrôle -
(Dominance)
Donc - (Therefore)
Données - (Information;
data)
Donner - (Give)
Donneur - (Donor)
Dormir - (Sleep, to)
Dorsal - (Dorsal)
Dos - (Back)
Dos - (Back)
Dos de la main - (Back of
the hand)
Dos du pied - (Back of the
feet)
Dose - (Dosage)

Dose - (Dose)
Dose de maintenance, demaintien - (Maintenance dose)
Dossier médical - (Clinical history)
Dossier médical - (Medical File)
Doucement - (Slowly)
Douleur - (Pain)
Douleur - (Pain)
Doute - (Doubt)
douves - (flukes)
Doux(ce - (Sweet)
Doxycycline - (Doxycycline)
Doyen - (Dean)
Drainage - (Drainage)
Drainer - (Drain)
Drépanocyte - (Sickle cell)
Drépanocytose - (Sickle cell disease)
Drogué(e - (Drug addict)
Drogue(s - (Drug(s))
Drogues intraveineuses - (Intravenous drugs)
Droit(e - (Right)
Duodénite - (Duodenitis)
Duodénoscopie - (Duodenoscopy)
Duodénum - (Duodenum)
Dur(e - (Hard)
Durant - (During)
Duvet - (Hair on the body, face)
Dysarthrie - (Dysarthria)
Dyscrasie - (Dyscrasia)
Dysenterie - (Dysentery)
Dysenterie amibienne - (Amoebic dysentery)
Dysesthésie - (Dysesthesia)
Dysfonctionnement - (Dysfunction)
Dysgénésie - (Dysgenesis)
Dyskinésie - (Dyskinesia)
Dysménorrhée - (Dysmenorrhea)
Dyspareunie - (Dispareunia; painful sex)
Dyspepsie - (Dyspepsia)
Dysphagie - (Dysphagia)
Dysphonie - (Dysphonia)
Dysplasie - (Dysplasia)
Dyspnée - (Dyspnea)
Dyspnéique - (Dyspneic)
Dystocie - (Dystocia)
Dystrophie - (Dystrophy)
Dysurie - (Dysuria)

~ E ~

Eau - (Water)
Eau bouillie - (Boiled water)
Eau de source - (Underground water)
Eau distillée - (Distilled

water)
Eau douce, potable - (Fresh water)
Eau oxygénée - (Oxygenated water)
Eau potable - (Drinking water)
Eau résiduelle - (Residual water)
Écailleux(se - (Scaly; flaky)
Ecchymose - (Ecchymosis; bruise)
Echange - (Exchange)
Echantillon - (Sample)
échantillon de sang - (blood sample)
Échec - (Failure)
Echo - (Echo)
Echocardiographie - (Echocardiography)
Echographie - (Echography)
Éclaircissement - (Clarification)
Eclampsie - (Eclampsia)
Écographie - (Ultrasound)
Écographie diagnostique - (Ultrasound, diagnostic)
École de médecine - (Medical school)
Economie - (Economy)
Écourter - (Shorten, to)
Écran - (Screen)

Ectasie - (Ectasia)
Ectopie - (Ectopy)
Eczéma - (Eczema)
Education - (Education)
Education sanitaire - (Health education)
Education sexuelle - (Sexual education)
Effet - (Effect)
Effet adverse - (Adverse effect)
Effet collatéral - (Collateral effect)
Effet toxique - (Toxic effect)
Effets nocifs - (Adverse effects)
Effets tardifs - (Delayed effects)
Efficace - (Effective)
Effort - (Effort)
Effusion - (Effusion)
Egal - (Equal)
Égratignure - (Scratch)
Éjaculation - (Ejaculation)
Éjaculer - (Ejaculate)
Élancement - (Stabbing pain; shooting pain)
Élastique - (Elastic)
Electricité - (Electricity)
Electrocardiogramme - (Electrocardiogram)
ElectroencéphalogrammeEE

G - (Electroencephalogram; EEG)

Electrolyte - (Electrolyte)

Electromyogramme EMG - (Electromyogram; EMG)

Elément - (Element)

Éléphantiasis - (Elephantiasis)

Elimination - (Elimination)

Eliminer - (Eliminate)

Elixir - (Elixir)

Embolie - (Embolism)

Embolie cérébrale - (Cerebral embolism)

Embolisme - (Embolism)

Embrasser - (Kiss, to)

Embryologie - (Embryology)

Embryon - (Embryo)

Émétique - (Emetic)

Éminence métatarsienne - (Metatarsal)

Émollient - (Emollient)

Emotion - (Emotion)

Emouvoir, émotionner - (Shock, to)

Empêcher - (Block, to; prevent, to)

Emphysémateux - (Emphysematous)

Emphysème - (Emphysema)

Empirer - (Worsen, to)

Empoisonnement - (Poisoning)

Empoisonner - (Poison, to)

Empreintes digitales - (Fingerprint)

Empyème - (Empyema)

Emulsion - (Emulsion)

En avant, progresser - (Ahead)

En capsule - (Encapsulated)

En haut - (Above)

En mauvais état - (In bad shape)

En plus - (In addition)

En relation avec l'épiphyse - (Epiphysis, in relation to)

En séquence - (Sequential)

Énanthème - (Enanthem; rash on mucous membranes)

Enceinte - (Pregnancy)

Enceinte - (Pregnant)

Enceinte - (Pregnant)

Enceinte pour la première fois - (Primigravida)

Encéphale - (Encephalus; brain)

Encéphalite - (Encephalitis)

Encéphalomyélite - (Encephalomyelitis)

Encéphalopathie - (Encephalopathy)

Enclume - (Anvil; incus)

Encoprésie - (Encopresis)

Endaortite - (Endaortitis)

Endartériectomie - (Endarterectomy)
Endartérite - (Endarteritis)
Endémie - (Endemic)
Endémique - (Endemic)
Endocarde - (Endocardium)
Endocardite - (Endocarditis)
Endocrine - (Endocrine)
Endocrinologie - (Endocrinology)
Endogène - (Endogenous)
Endomètre - (Endometrium)
Endométriose - (Endometriosis)
Endométrite - (Endometritis)
Endormi(e - (Drowsy)
Endoscopie - (Endoscopy)
Endothélium - (Endothelium)
Endotoxine - (Endotoxin)
Endotoxique - (Endotoxic)
Enéma, lavement - (Enema)
Energie - (Energy)
Enfance - (Childhood)
Enfance - (Infancy)
Enfant prématuré - (Infant, premature)
Enflé (e - (Inflamed)
Enflé (e - (Swollen)
Enfler - (Swell, to)
Engourdi(e), endormi(e -

(Numbed; sedated)
engrais minéraux - (fertiliser)
Enlever, retirer - (Remove, to)
Enregistrer - (Register, to)
Enrhumé - (Cold; upper respiratory infection)
Enrhumé - (Sick with a cold)
Enrouement - (Hoarseness)
Ensanglanté(e - (Bloody)
Entassement - (Overcrowded housing; stacking; heaping; accumulation)
Entendre - (Hear, to)
Entérite - (Enteritis)
entérite - (enteritis)
Entérobiase - (Enterobiasis)
Entérocolite - (Enterocolitis)
Entéropathie - (Enteropathy)
Entérotoxine - (Enterotoxin)
Entérovirus - (Enterovirus)
Entorse - (Sprain)
Entorse - (Sprain)
Entorse, distorsion - (Distortion)
Entourage, environnement - (Surrounding; environment of)
Énurésie - (Enuresis)

Envahisseur - (Invador)

Environnement - (Environment)

Environnement - (Environment)

Environnement contrôlé - (Environmental control)

Environnement de travail - (Work environment)

Envoi - (Shipping)

enzootique - (enzootic)

Éosinophile - (Eosinophilic)

Éosinophilie - (Eosinophilia)

Épaississement, engraisser - (Swelling)

Épanchement liquide synovial - (Synovial effusion)

Épanchement pleural - (Pleural effusion)

Epaule - (Shoulder)

Éperon sous-calcanéen - (Spur)

Épicondylite - (Epicondylitis)

Épidémie - (Epidemic)

Épidémiologie - (Epidemiology)

Épidémique - (Epidemic)

Épiderme - (Epidermis)

Épidermique - (Epidermic)

Épididyme - (Epididymo)

Épidural - (Epidural)

Épigastralgie -

(Epigastralgia)

Épigastre - (Epigastrium)

Épiglotte - (Epiglottis)

Épilepsie - (Epilepsy)

Épileptique - (Epileptic)

Épine bifide - (Spina bifida)

Épine dorsale - (Spine)

Épiphyse - (Epiphysis)

Épisiotomie - (Episiotomy)

Épisode - (Episode)

Épistaxis - (Epistaxis)

Épithélioma - (Epithelioma)

Épithélium - (Epithelium)

épizootie - (epizootic)

Epouiller - (Delouse)

Époux/ Épouse - (Spouse)

Épreinte - (Urge; straining; push)

Éprouvette - (Manometer)

Épuisé (e - (Exhausted)

Équilibre - (Equilibrium)

Équipe - (Team)

Équivalent - (Equivalent)

éradiquer - (eradicate)

Érection - (Erection)

Ergothérapie - (Ergotherapy)

Erreur - (Error)

Erreur, défaillance - (Failure)

Éructation, faire des rots - (Eructation; Burp; Belch)

Éruption - (Eruption)

Érysipèle - (Erysipelas)

Érythème - (Erythema)
Érythrocyte - (Erythrocyte)
Érythropoïèse - (Erythropoiesis)
Escarre - (Eschar; scab)
Éscherichia Coli - (Escherichia coli)
Espèce - (Species)
Espérance de vie - (Life expectancy)
Esprit - (Spirit)
Essai, pratique, test - (Test; essay)
Estomac - (Stomach)
estomac - (stomach)
Estrogène - (Estrogen)
État - (State)
État d'esprit - (Mood)
État de santé - (State of health)
État de veille, surveillance - (Wakefulness)
État végétatif - (Vegetative state)
Été - (Summer)
Éternuement - (Sneeze)
Éternuer - (Sneeze, to)
Éthique - (Ethic)
Éthique médicale - (Medical ethic)
Étiologie - (Etiology)
Étiologique - (Etiologic)

Étouffement - (Asphyxia)
Étouffement, noyade - (Drowning)
Étouffer - (Asphyxiate)
Etre - (Be, to)
Étudiant en médecine - (Medical student)
Euphorie - (Euphoria)
Évacuation - (Evacuation)
Évacuer - (Evacuate)
Évagination - (Evagination)
Évaluation - (Evaluation)
Evanouissement - (Faint)
Evanouissement - (Faint)
Eveillé - (Awake)
Évènement - (Event)
Éventail thérapeutique - (Window, therapeutic)
Évolution - (Evolution)
Exacerbation - (Exacerbation)
Examen - (Exam)
Examen oral - (Oral exam)
Examen physique - (Physical exam)
Examiner - (Examine, to)
Examiner, ausculter - (Examine, to; recognize, to)
Exanthème - (Exanthema)
Excès de gras dans les matières fécales - (Steatorrhoea)

Excessif (ive - (Excessive)
Excipient, substance -
(Excipient)
Excitation - (Excitement;
arousal)
Excrément - (Excrement)
excréments - (faeces)
Excrétion - (Excretion)
Exemple - (Example)
Exercer - (Practice)
Exercice physique -
(Physical exercise)
Exfoliation - (Exfoliation)
Exhaler - (Exhale)
Exocrine - (Exocrine)
Exogène - (Exogenous)
Exophtalmie -
(Exophthalmos)
Exophtalmie - (Proptosis)
Expectorant - (Expectorant)
Expectoration -
(Expectoration)
Expérience - (Experience)
Expérimental(e -
(Experimental)
Expiration - (Expiration)
Expirer - (Expire)
Expirer, périmer - (Expire, to
(medication))
Exploration - (Exploration)
Exposé - (Exposed)
Exposition - (Exposition)
Expulser - (Expel)

Exstrophie - (Extrophy)
Extension - (Extension)
Extérieur - (Exterior)
Extérioriser - (Externalize)
Exterminer - (Exterminate)
Externe - (External)
Extirpation - (Extirpation;
removal)
Extirper - (Extirpate;
remove)
Extraction - (Extraction)
Extraction dentaire -
(Extraction, dental)
Extraire - (Extract, to)
Extrasystole - (Extrasystole)
Extra-utérin - (Extrauterine)
Extravasation -
(Extravasation)
Extravasculaire -
(Extravascular)
Extrême - (Extreme)
Extrémité - (Limb)
Extrémité inférieure -
(Lower limb)
Extrémité supérieure -
(Upper limb)

~ F ~

Face antérieure - (Backside;
reverse side)
Facial(e - (Facial)

Faciès - (Facies)
Facile - (Easy)
Facteur - (Factor)
Facteur de risque - (Risk factor)
Facture - (Invoice; bill)
Facultatif (ive - (Facultative)
Faculté de médecine - (Medical school)
Faible - (Weak)
Faiblesse, débilité - (Weakness)
Faim - (Hunger)
Faire - (Do, to; make, to)
Faire mal - (Feel pain, to)
Faire sa toilette - (Clean up)
Faire une inspection - (Inspect, to)
Faire une transfusion - (Transfuse)
Faisceau - (Fascicle; bundle)
Fait - (Done; made; fact; data)
Fait mal - (Hurt)
Falciforme - (Falciform; sickle shaped)
Falsification - (Adulteration)
Falsifié(e - (Adulterated)
Familier - (Relative, a; familiar)
Famille - (Family)
Famine - (Famine)

Fasciculation, contraction desfibres musculaires involontaire - (Fasciculation; involuntary contraction of muscle fibers)
Fasciole - (Fasciola; genus of flukes, a)
Fasciole hépatique - (Fasciola hepatica; liver fluke)
Fatal (e - (Fatal)
Fatigue - (Fatigue)
Fatigue - (Fatigue)
Fatigué(e - (Tired)
Fatigué, suffoqué - (Fatigued; tired)
Faux - (false)
Faux dents - (False teeth)
Fébrile - (Febrile; feverish)
Fécal - (Fecal)
Fécalome - (Fecaloma; tumor of impacted feces)
Fèces - (Feces)
Fécondation - (Fertilization; fecundation)
Féconder - (Fertilize, to; fecundate, to)
Fécondité - (Fertile; fecund)
Feindre, faire semblant - (Pretend, to)
Féminin (e - (Feminine)
Femme - (Woman)

Femmes en couches - (Parturient; woman in labor)
Fémur - (Femur)
Fenêtre - (Window)
Fénitöine - (Phenytoin)
Fer - (Iron)
Fermé (e - (Closed)
Fermer - (Close, to)
Fertile - (Fertile)
Fertilité - (Fertility)
Fesse - (Buttock (butt))
Fesse - (Gluteus; buttock)
Feuille - (Leaf; sheet of paper)
Feuille de route clinique - (Health form)
Fibrillation - (Fibrillation)
Fibrillation auriculaire - (Atrial fibrillation)
Fibrillation ventriculaire - (Ventricular fibrillation)
Fibrine - (Fibrin)
Fibrinogène - (Fibrinogen)
Fibrinolyse - (Fibrinolysis)
Fibrinopénie, manque defibrine - (Fibrinopenia)
Fibrome - (Fibroma)
Fibromyosite - (Fibromyositis)
Fibrose - (Fibrosis)
Fibrose kystique - (Cystic fibrosis)
Fibrose pulmonaire -

(Pulmonary fibrosis)
Fibule, agrafe, péroné - (Fibula)
Fière rhumatismale - (Rheumatic fever)
Fièvre - (Fever)
fièvre - (fever)
Fièvre jaune - (Yellow fever)
Fièvre typhoïde - (Typhoid fever)
Fiévreux(se - (Febrile)
Fiévreux(se - (Febrile, feverish)
Fille - (Daughter)
Fils - (Son)
Filtration - (Filtration)
Filtre - (Filter)
Fin - (End)
Fiole, ampoule - (Vial)
Fissure - (Fissure)
Fissure - (Incision)
Fistule - (Fistula)
Fixation - (Fixation)
Flasque - (Flaccid; limp)
Flatulence - (Flatulence)
Flegme - (Phlegm; mucus)
Flexion - (Flexion)
Flore - (Flora)
Flore intestinale normale - (Normal intestinal flora)
Fluctuer - (Fluctuate)
Fluide - (Fluid)
Flux - (Discharge; drainage;

flow)
Flux sanguin - (Blood flow)
flystrike - (flystrike)
Fœtal - (Fetal)
Fœtographie, radiographie
dufœtus - (Fetography; fetal
radiograph)
Fœtométrie, mesure du
fœtus - (Fetometry;
estimation of fetal size)
Fœtoprotéine -
(Fetoprotein)
Fœtus - (Fetus)
foetus - (foetus)
Foie - (Liver)
Follicule - (Follicle)
Folliculite - (Folliculitis)
Fomites - (Fomites)
Foncé (e - (Dark)
Fonction - (Function)
Fond - (Fundus; base;
bottom)
Fond - (Fundus; base;
bottom)
Fond d'œil - (Fundus of the
eye)
Fongicide - (Fungicide)
Fongus - (Fungus)
Fongus, champignon -
(Fungus)
Fontanelle - (Fontanel)
Fontanelle antérieure -

(Anterior fontanel)
Fontanelle postérieure -
(Posterior fontanel)
Foramen, orifice -
(Foramen; orifice)
Forceps - (Forceps)
Formation de calcul dans
l'urètre - (Stone, urinary)
Forme - (Form; shape)
Fosse - (Fossa)
Fosse nasale - (Nostril)
Fosse septique - (Tank,
septic)
Fou - (Insane)
fourbure - (laminitis)
Fourmillement - (Pins and
needles, sensation of; ant
hill)
Foyer pour personnes âgées
- (Nursing home)
Fraction - (Fraction; part)
Fracture - (Fracture)
Fraise - (Strawberry)
Frémir - (Fremitus)
Fréquence - (Frequency;
rate)
Fréquence cardiaque -
(Heart rate)
Fréquence respiratoire -
(Respiratory rate)
Frère/ Sœur - (Brother /
sister)

Frigidité - (Frigidity)
Frisson - (Shiver)
Froid (e - (Cold)
Front - (Forehead)
Frontal(e - (Frontal)
Frottement - (Rub; friction)
Frotter - (Rub, to)
Frottis - (Smear)
frottis de sang - (blood smear)
Frottis vaginal - (Vaginal smear)
Fugace - (Fleeting)
Fulminant (e - (Fulminant)
Fumer - (Smoke, to)
Fumeur - (Smoker)
Fumigation - (Fumigation)
Fumiger - (Fumigate, to)
Furoncle - (Carbuncle)
Furoncle - (Furuncle)
Furoncle - (Furuncle)
Futur - (Future)

~ G ~

Gagner du poids - (Gain weight)
Gaine - (Sheath)
Galacthorrée - (Galactorrhea)
Gale - (Scabies)
Gale - (Scabies)

Gammaglobuline - (Gamma globulin)
Ganglion - (Ganglion)
Ganglion - (Ganglion)
Ganglion lymphatique - (Lymphatic ganglion)
ganglionnaire - (lymph node)
Gangrène - (Gangrene)
Gant - (Glove)
Gants chirurgicaux - (Surgical gloves)
Garçon - (Male; man)
Garçon / Fille - (Child)
Gargarisme, faire des gargarismes - (Gargle)
Gastralgie - (Gastralgia; stomach ache)
Gastrite - (Gastritis)
Gastro-duodénal - (Gastroduodenal)
Gastro-entérite - (Gastroenteritis)
gastro-entérite - (gastro-enteritis)
Gastro-entérocolite - (Gastroenterocolitis)
Gastro-intestinal - (Gastrointestinal)
Gastro-œesophage - (Gastroesophageal)
Gastroscopie - (Gastroscopy)

Gauche - (Left)

Gaze - (Gauze)

Gazoline, essence - (Gasoline)

Gelée - (Jelly)

Gencive - (Gingiva; gums)

Gencive - (Gum)

Gène - (Gene)

Gène, dérangement - (Discomfort; nuisance)

Général - (General)

Genèse - (Genesis; origin)

Génétique - (Genetic)

Génital - (Genital)

Génitaux - (Genitals)

Génito-urinaire - (Urogenital)

Génome - (Genome)

Génotype - (Genotype)

Genou - (Knee)

Genre - (Gender)

Genre féminin - (Female)

Genre masculin - (Male)

Gentamicine - (Gentamycin)

Gériatrie - (Geriatrics)

Gériatrique - (Geriatric)

Germe - (Germ)

Germicide - (Germicide)

gésier - (gizzard)

Gestation, grossesse - (Gestation)

Gestion ou contrôle de la

maladie - (Management, illness)

Gestose - (Gestosis)

Giardia - (Giardia)

Giardiase, lambiose - (Giardiasis)

Gingivite - (Gingivitis)

Gingivorragie - (Gingivorrhagia)

Glace - (Ice)

Glande - (Gland)

Glande - (Gland)

glande - (gland)

glande thyroïde - (thyroid gland)

Glandes endocrines - (Endocrine glands)

Glandes exocrines - (Exocrine glands)

Glandes salivaires - (Salivary glands)

Glaucome - (Glaucoma)

globules - (blood cell)

Globules blancs - (White blood cell)

Globules rouges - (Red blood cell)

Glomérulaire - (Glomerular)

Glomérulonéphrite - (Glomerulonephritis)

Glossalgie - (Glossalgia)

Glossite - (Glossitis)

Glotte - (Glottis)
Glucocorticoïde - (Glucocorticoid)
Glucopénie - (Glycopenia)
Glucose - (Glucose)
Glucoside - (Glucoside)
Glucourie - (Glycosuria)
Glycémie - (Glycemia)
Glycémie - (Glycemia)
Glycogène - (Glycogen)
Goitre - (Goiter)
Goitre exophtalmique - (Exophthalmic goiter)
Gonade - (Gonad)
Gonadique - (Gonadal)
Gonadotrophine - (Gonadotropin)
Gonflement - (Swelling)
Gonorrhée - (Gonorrhea)
Gorge - (Throat)
Goût - (Taste)
Goutte - (Drop; drip)
Graisse - (Fat)
Gram- négatif - (Gram negative)
Gramme - (Gram)
Gramme - (Gram)
Gram-positif - (Gram positive)
Grand - (Large)
Grandeur - (Size)
Grandir, croître - (Grow, to)
Grand-père, grand- mère -
(Grandfather)
Granule - (Granule)
Granulocytopénie - (Granulocytopenia)
Grappe - (Cluster; bunch)
Gratter - (Scratch, to)
Gratuit - (Free)
Grave - (Acute)
Grave - (Serious)
Greffe - (Graft)
Grincement des dents, bruxisme - (Grinding one's teeth; bruxism)
Grippe, rhume - (Cold, a)
Grippe, Rhume - (Flu; influenza)
Gris - (Grey)
Gros intestin - (Intestine, large)
Gros orteil - (Big toe)
Gros(se), épais(se - (Thick)
Gros, grosse, obèse - (Fat; obese)
Grossesse compliquée - (Complicated pregnancy)
Grossesse ectopique - (Ectopic pregnancy)
Grossesse multiple, gémellaire - (Multiple pregnancy)
Grosseur - (Thickness)
Grossir, engraisser - (Gain weight, to)

Groupe - (Group; type)
Groupe sanguin - (Blood type)
Guêpe - (Wasp)
Guérir - (Heal, to)
Guérison - (Treatment)
Guérissable - (Curable)
Gynécologie - (Gynecology)
Gynécologue - (Gynecologist)
Gynécomastie - (Gynecomastia)

~ H ~

Habitude - (Custom; habit)
Habitude - (Habit)
Habitué(e - (Accustomed)
Habituel - (Habitual)
Haematocolpos - (Hematocolpos; retained menstruation)
Haleine - (Breath; strength)
Halètement - (Panting; gasping)
Halitose - (Halitosis)
Hallucination - (Hallucination)
Hanche - (Hip)
Handicapé - (Disabilities, person with)

Handicapé - (Disabled; handicapped)
Harcèlement sexuel - (Sexual harassment)
Hauteur - (Height)
Hebdomadaire - (Weekly)
Helminthe - (Parasitic worm)
helminthes - (helminths)
Helminthiase - (Parasitic worm infections)
Hématémèse - (Hematemesis; vomiting blood)
Hématie - (Red blood cells)
Hématocrite - (Red blood cell count)
Hématologique - (Hematologic)
Hématome - (Hematoma)
Hématome sud dural - (Subdural hematoma)
Hématopoïèse - (Hematopoiesis)
Hématurie - (Hematuria; blood in the urine)
Hémiatrophie - (Hemiatrophy; atrophy of half)
Hémicrânie - (Hemicrania)
Hémiparésie - (Hemiparesis)
Hémiplégie - (Hemiplegia)

Hémiplégique - (Hemiplegic)
Hémisphère - (Hemisphere)
Hémithorax - (Hemithorax)
Hémo thorax -
(Hemothorax)
Hémo-concentration -
(Hemoconcentration)
Hémoculture - (Blood
culture)
Hémodialyse -
(Hemodialysis)
Hémoglobine -
(Hemoglobin)
Hémoglobinopathie -
(Hemoglobinopathy)
Hémogramme -
(Hemogram)
Hémolyse - (Hemolysis)
Hémophilie - (Hemophilia)
Hémoptysie - (Hemoptysis)
Hémorragie - (Hemorrhage)
Hémorragie - (Hemorrhage)
hémorragie - (haemorrhage
)
Hémorragie cérébrale -
(Cerebral hemorrhage)
Hémorragie cérébrale -
(Hemorrhagic stroke;
cerebral vascular accident)
Hémorragie du larynx -
(Laryngorrhagia;
hemorrhage from the
larynx)

Hémorragie intestinale -
(Enterorrhagia; intestinal
hemorrhage)
Hémorragique -
(Hemorrhagic)
Hémorroïde - (Hemorrhoid)
Hémostase - (Hemostasis)
Héparine - (Heparin)
Hépatique - (Hepatic)
Hépatite - (Hepatitis)
Hépatite aiguë - (Acute
hepatitis)
Hépatite fulminante -
(Fulminant hepatitis)
Hépato biliaire -
(Hepatobiliary)
Hépato toxine -
(Hepatotoxicity)
Hépatologie - (Hepatology)
Hépatomégalie -
(Hepatomegaly; enlarged
liver)
Hépato-splénomégalie -
(Hepatosplenomegaly;
enlarged liver and spleen)
Héréditaire - (Hereditary)
Héritage - (Inheritance;
heredity, to)
Héritage dominant -
(Dominant characteristic)
Héritage récessif,
héritagecytoplasmique -
(Recessive characteristic)

Hernie - (Hernia; herniatiom)
Hernie étranglée - (Hernia, strangulated)
Hernie hiatale - (Hernia, hiatal)
Hernie inguinale - (Hernia, inguinal)
Hernie ombilicale - (Hernia, umbilical)
Herniographie - (Herniorrhaphy; hernia repair)
Herpangine - (Herpangina)
Herpès - (Herpes)
Herpès génital - (Genital herpes)
Herpès zoster, zona - (Herpes zoster)
Hétérogène - (Heterogeneous)
Hétérosexualité - (Heterosexuality)
Hétérosexuel - (Heterosexual)
Heure - (Hour)
Heure de consultation - (Working hours)
Heure de visite - (Visiting hours)
Hiatus - (Hiatus)
Hier - (Yesterday)

Hile - (Hilum)
Hirsutisme - (Hirsutism)
Histologie - (Histology)
Histologique - (Histologist)
Histoplasmose - (Histoplasmosis)
Homéostasie - (Homeostasis)
Homicide - (Homicide)
Homme - (Man)
Homologue - (Homologous)
Homosexualité - (Homosexuality)
Homosexuel - (Homosexual)
Homozygote - (Homozygote)
Hôpital - (Hospital)
Hôpital - (Hospital)
Hôpital général - (Hospital, general)
Hôpital militaire - (Hospital, military)
Hôpital municipal - (Hospital, city)
Hôpital pédiatrique - (Hospital, children's)
Hôpital rural - (Hospital, rural)
Hoquet - (Hiccups)
Horizontal - (Horizontal)
Hormonal - (Hormonal)
Hormone - (Hormone)

hormone - (hormone)
Hors de la vessie -
(Extravesical)
Hors du vagin, extra-vaginal
- (Extravaginal)
Hospitalisation -
(Hospitalization)
Hospitaliser - (Hospitalize)
hôtes - (hosts)
Huitième - (Eighth)
Humain - (Human)
Humérus - (Humerus)
Humeur - (Body fluid;
humor; mood)
Humeur aqueuse -
(Aqueous humor)
Humoral- relatifs aux
humeurs du corps -
(Humoral; body fluids,
pertaining to)
Hydratation - (Hydration)
Hydrater - (Hydrate)
Hydro adénite -
(Hidradenitis)
Hydrocéphalie -
(Hydrocephaly)
Hydronéphrose -
(Hydronephrosis)
Hydrophile - (Hydrophilic)
Hydrophobie -
(Hydrophobia)
Hydropisie - (Hydropsy)
Hydro-pnéumothorax -

(Hydropneumothorax)
Hydrosalpinx -
(Hydrosalpinx)
Hydrosoluble - (Water
soluble)
Hydrothorax - (Hydrothorax)
Hygiène - (Hygiene)
Hygiène buccale - (Oral
hygiene)
Hygiénique - (Hygienic)
Hymen - (Hymen)
Hyper - (Hyper)
Hyper acidité -
(Hyperacidity)
Hyper réactivité -
(Hyperreactivity)
Hyper sécrétion -
(Hypersecretion)
Hyper ventilation -
(Hyperventilation)
Hyperactivité -
(Hyperactivity)
Hyperbilirrubinémie -
(Hyperbilirubinemia)
hypercalcémie -
(Hypercalcemia)
Hypercholestérolémie -
(Hypercholesterolemia)
Hypercinésie -
(Hyperkinesia)
Hyperémie - (Hyperemia)
Hyperesthésie -
(Hyperesthesia)

Hyperfibrinémie -
(Hyperfibrinemia)
Hyperglycémie -
(Hyperglycemia)
Hyperhydrose -
(Hyperhidrosis)
Hyperlipidémie -
(Hyperlipidemia)
Hyperménorrhée -
(Menorraghia)
Hypermétropie - (Hyperopia
(farsightedness))
Hypermétropie - (Hyperopia
(farsightedness))
Hyperplasie - (Hyperplasia)
Hyperplasie - (Hyperplasia)
Hyperpnée - (Hyperpnea)
Hyperpotassémie -
(Hyperkalemia)
Hypersalivation - (Drooling)
Hypersensibilité -
(Hypersensitivity)
Hypertendu -
(Hypertensive)
Hypertenseur -
(Hypertensive)
Hypertension -
(Hypertension (high blood
pressure))
Hyperthermie -
(Hyperthermia)
Hyperthermie -

(Hyperthermia)
Hyperthyroïdie -
(Hyperthyroidism)
Hypertonie - (Hypertonia)
Hypertrophie -
(Hypertrophy)
Hyperuricémie -
(Hyperuricemia)
Hypervolémie -
(Hypervolemia)
Hypo-activité - (Hypoactive)
Hypochondriaque -
(Hypochondriac)
Hypochondrie -
(Hypochondria)
Hypocinésie - (Hypokinesia)
Hypoderme - (Hypodermis)
Hypodermique -
(Hypodermic)
Hypofonction -
(Hypofunction
(insufficiency))
Hypoglosse - (Hypoglossal)
Hypoglycémie -
(Hypoglycemia)
Hypoglycémique -
(Hypoglycemic)
Hypogonadisme -
(Hypogonadism (low
testosterone))
Hypoperfusion -
(Hypoperfusion)

Hypophysaire - (Hypophysis, of the; pituitary, of the)
Hypophyse - (Hypophysis; pituitary gland)
Hypopituitarisme - (Hypopituitarism)
Hypopotassémie - (Hypokalemia)
Hyporéflectivité - (Hyporeflexia)
Hyposalivation - (Xerostomia (dry mouth))
Hyposodé - (Hyponatremia)
Hypotendu (e - (Hypotensive)
Hypotension - (Hypotension (low blood pressure))
hypotension - (Hypotensive)
Hypothalamus - (Hypothalamus)
Hypothermie - (Hypothermia)
Hypotonie - (Hypotonia)
Hypotyroïdisme - (Hypothyroidism)
Hypoventilation - (Hypoventilation (respiratory depression))
Hypovitaminose - (Avitaminosis)
Hypovolémie - (Hypovolemia)

Hypoxie - (Hypoxia)
Hypoxique - (Hypoxic)
hystérectomie - (Hysterectomy)
Hystérie - (Hysteria)
Hystérique - (Hysterical)

~ I ~

Iatrogenie - (Iatrogen)
Iatrogénique - (Iatrogenic)
Iatrogènique - (Iatrogenic)
Ichthyose - (Ichtyosis)
Ictérique, qui a la jaunisse - (Jaundiced)
Idée identique - (Idea, same)
Identification - (Identification)
Idiopathique - (Idiopathic)
Idiosyncrasie - (Idiosyncrasy)
Ignorer - (Ignore; unaware of, to be)
Iléite - (Ileitis)
Iléon - (Ileum)
Iléon - (Ileum)
Iliaque - (Iliac)
Image - (Image)
Imbécile - (Imbecile)
Immature - (Immature)
Immobilisation -

(Immobilization)
immunisation -
(Immunization)
Immunité - (Immunity)
Immuno-dépression -
(Immunosuppression)
Immunologie -
(Immunology)
Immunosuppresseur -
(Immunosuppressant)
Impalpable - (Impalpable)
Imparfait - (Imperfect)
Impénétrable -
(Impenetrable)
Imperforé(e -
(Unperforated)
Impétigo - (Impetigo)
Implanter - (Implant, to)
Implication - (Implication)
Importance - (Importance)
Importance - (Importance)
imprégnation -
(Impregnation)
Imprégner - (Impregnate,
to)
Improbable - (Improbable;
unlikely)
Impuissance - (Impotence)
Impulsion, élan - (Impulse)
Impur (e - (Impure)
Impureté - (Impurity)
In situ, sur le terrain - (In

situ)
In vitro - (In vitro)
In vivo - (In vivo)
Inaccessible - (Inaccessible)
Inactif (ive - (Inactive)
Inadéquat (e - (Inadequate)
Inanition - (Inanition)
Incapable - (Disabled)
Incapable - (Incapable)
Incapacité - (Disability)
Incarcération -
(Incarceration)
Incendie - (Fire)
Incidence - (Incidence)
Incisif (ive - (Incisive)
Incision - (Slit; crack; split)
Incliné - (Inclined)
Inclure - (Include, to)
Inclus - (Included)
Incohérent - (Incoherent)
Incompatible -
(Incompatible)
Incompétent -
(Incompetent)
Inconscient - (Unconscious)
Incontinence -
(Incontinence)
Incontinent - (Incontinent)
Incoordination - (Lack of
coordination)
Incubation - (Incubation)
incubation - (incubation)

incubation - (incubation)
Incurable - (Incurable)
Indemne - (Unharmed)
Indésirable - (Unwanted)
Index - (Index finger)
Indication - (Indication;
instruction; order)
Indigeste - (Indigestible)
Indigestion - (Indigestion)
Indigestion - (Indigestion)
Indiqué - (Indicated;
specified)
indiquer - (Indicate, to;
prescribe, to)
Indirect (e - (Indirect)
Indispensable -
(Indispensable)
Individuel - (Individual)
Indolore - (Painless)
Induction - (Induction)
Inefficace - (Inefficient)
Inerte - (Inert)
Inertie - (Inertia)
Infantile - (Children's;
childhood)
Infarctus - (Infarct)
Infecté (e - (Infected)
Infecter - (Infect, to)
Infectieux (se - (Infectious)
Infection - (Infection)
infection - (infection)
Infection acquise dans la
communauté - (Infection,

community acquired)
Infection aiguë - (Infection,
acute)
Infection au contact minime
- (Infection, minimal
contact)
Infection chronique -
(Infection, chronic)
Infection opportuniste -
(Infection, opportunistic)
Infection sous clinique -
(Infection, subclinical)
infertiles - (infertile)
Infertilité - (Infertility)
Infestation - (Infestation)
Infiltration - (Infiltration)
Infiltré (e - (Infiltrated)
Infirmerie - (Infirmary)
Infirmier(ière - (Nurse)
Inflammation -
(Inflammation)
inflammation -
(inflammation)
Inflammation d'une valvule
- (Valvulitis)
Inflammation de l'épiglotte -
(Epiglottitis)
Inflammation des jointures -
(Sacroilitis)
Inflammation du jéjunum -
(Jejunitis)
Influenza - (Influenza)
Information - (Information)

Infra claviculaire - (Infraclavicular)
Infrarouge - (Infrared)
Infrastructure sanitaire - (Health infrastructure)
Infusion - (Infusion)
ingérer - (Ingest; consume)
Ingestion de médicament - (Ingestion of medication)
Inguinal - (Inguinal)
Ingurgité(e - (Ingurgitated)
Inhalateur - (Inhaler)
Inhalation - (Inhalation; breath)
Inhaler - (Inhale, to)
Inhibition - (Inhibition)
Injecter - (Inject, to)
Injection - (Injection)
Injection sous-cutanée - (Injection, subcutaneous)
Inné - (Innate; inborn)
Innervation - (Innervation)
Innervé (e - (Innervated)
Inoculation - (Inoculation)
Inodore - (Odorless)
Inopérable - (Inoperable)
Inorganique - (Inorganic)
Inotropique - (Inotropic)
Insecte - (Insect)
insecticide - (insecticide)
Insensible - (Insensitive)
Insérer - (Insert, to)

Insertion - (Insertion)
Insolation - (Insolation)
Insoluble - (Insoluble)
Insomniaque - (Insomnia)
Inspection - (Inspection)
Inspiration - (Inhale)
Instable - (Unstable)
Instillation - (Instillation)
Instrumentale - (Instrumental)
Insuffisance - (Insufficiency)
Insuffisance cardiaque - (Heart failure)
Insuline - (Insulin)
Insupportable - (Unbearable; intolerable)
Intelligence - (Intelligence)
Intensité - (Intensity)
Intention - (Intention)
Interaction - (Interaction)
Interaction des médicaments - (Interaction of medications)
Intercostal - (Intercostal)
Intercurrent - (Intercurrent)
Interdit (e - (Prohibited)
Interférence - (Interference)
Intermédiaire - (Intermediary)
Intermittent - (Intermittent)
Interne - (Internal)

Interroger - (Question, to; interrogate)
Interrompre - (Interrupt, to)
Interstitiel - (Interstitial)
Intervalle - (Interval)
Intervention - (Intervention)
Intervention chirurgicale - (Intervention, surgical)
intervertébral - (Intervertebral)
Intervertir - (Reverse, to)
Intestin - (Intestine)
intestin - (intestine)
Intestin grêle - (Intestine, small)
Intestinale - (Intestinal)
Intolérance - (Intolerance)
Intoxication - (Intoxication; poisoning)
Intoxication alimentaire - (Food poisoning)
Intoxiqué (e - (Poisoned)
Intra-abdominal - (Intra abdominal)
Intracrânien - (Intracranial)
Intramusculaire - (Intramuscular)
Intraoculaire - (Intraocular)
Intra-utérin - (Intrauterine)
Intraveineux(se - (Intravenous)
Intrinsèque - (Intrinsic; inherent)

Introducteur - (Intubator)
Introduire - (Introduce, to)
Introduit - (Introitus)
Introflexion - (Introflection)
Intromission - (Intromission)
Introspection - (Introspection)
Intubation - (Intubation)
Invagination - (Invagination)
Involution - (Involution)
Iode - (Iodine)
Ionisation - (Ionization)
Iris - (Iris)
Iritis - (Iritis)
Irrégulier - (Irregular; erratic)
Irrigation - (Irrigation)
Irrigation sanguine - (Blood irrigation)
Irritant - (Irritant)
Irritation - (Irritation)
Irriter - (Irritate, to)
Ischémie - (Ischemia)
Ischémique - (Ischemic)
Isolement des patients - (Patient isolation)
Isolement du malade mental - (Confinement of mental patient)
isoler - (isolate)
Isoler, éloigner - (Isolate,

to)
Isotonique - (Isotonic)
Ivre - (Inebriated)
Ivrogne - (Drinker)
Ivrogne, soulard - (Drunk)

~ J ~

Jamais - (Never)
Jambe - (Leg)
Jaunâtre - (Yellowish)
Jaune - (Yellow)
Jaune d'œuf, bout(doigt -
(Fingertip)
Jaunisse - (Jaundice)
Jaunisse du nouveau-né -
(Jaundice, neonatal)
Jéjunum - (Jejunum)
Jetable - (Disposable)
Jeune - (Young person)
Jeûne - (Fast (go without
eating))
Jeunesse - (Youth)
Jointure des doigts -
(Knuckle)
Joue - (Cheek)
Joue - (Cheek)
Jour - (Day)
Jours au lit - (Days on bed
rest)
Jours d'hospitalisation -
(Hospital stay)
Jours de repos - (Days of
rest)
Jugulaire - (Jugular)
Jumeau - (Twin)
Jumeaux identiques -
(Identical twins)
Jumeaux, Jumelles - (Twins)
Jus - (Juice)
Jusqu'a - (Until)
Juxtaposition -
(Juxtaposition)

~ K ~

Kanamycine - (Kanamycin)
Kératine - (Keratin)
Kératinisée - (Keratinized)
Kératite - (Keratitis)
Kérato-conjonctivite -
(Keratoconjunctivitis)
Kératolytique - (Keratolytic)
Kératose - (Keratosis)
Kilo, kilogramme - (Kilo;
kilogram)
Kilocalorie - (Kilocalorie)
Kilomètre - (Kilometer)
Kwashiorkor - (Kwashiorkor)
Kyste - (Cyst)
kyste - (cyst)
kyste hydatique - (hydatid

cyst)
Kystique - (Cystic)

~ L ~

la chaleur - (heat)
La jugulaire - (jugular)
La pression artérielle -
(blood pressure)
La trachée - (trachea)
La vessie - (bladder)
Labial - (Labial)
Laboratoire - (Laboratory)
Labyrinthite - (Labyrinthitis)
Lacération - (Laceration)
Lactose - (Lactose)
Lait - (Milk)
Lait de mère - (Breast milk;
mother's milk)
Laitier - (Milk, pertaining to;
dairy product)
Lancette - (Lancet)
Langage - (Language;
speech)
Langue - (Language)
Langue - (Tongue)
Laparoscopie -
(Laparoscopy)
Laparotomie - (Laparotomy)
Large - (Wide)
Larme - (Tear)
Larve - (Larva)

larve - (larva)
Larves - (Larvae)
Laryngite - (Laryngitis)
Laryngoscope -
(Laryngoscope)
Laryngoscopie -
(Laryngoscopy)
Larynx - (Larynx)
Latence - (Latency)
Latéral - (Lateral)
Latrines - (Latrine)
latrines - (latrine)
Lavage des mains - (Hand
washing)
Lavement - (Lavage)
l'avortement - (abortion)
laxatif - (laxative)
Laxatif (ive - (Laxative)
Laxisme - (Laxity, laxness)
le stress - (stress)
Léger - (Light; slight;
gentle)
Léger(ère - (Light; mild;
low-grade)
Légèrement fiévreux - (Low
grade fever)
Légume - (Vegetable)
Lente, Lentilles - (Lens;
eyeglasses)
Lèpre - (Leprosy)
Lépreux - (Leper)
Lésion, blessure - (Lesion;
injury)

Léthargie - (Lethargy)
Leucémie - (Leukemia)
Leucocyte - (Leukocyte)
Leucocytose - (Leukocytosis)
Leucopénie - (Leukopenia)
Leucoplasie - (Leukoplasia)
Leucorrhée –pertes blanches - (Leukorrhea)
Lèvre - (Lip; labium)
Lèvres gercées - (Chapped lips)
Libido - (Libido)
Lichénification - (Lichenification)
Lidocaïne - (Lidocaine)
Lieu, endroit - (Place)
Ligament - (Ligament)
Ligature - (Ligation)
Ligature des trompes - (Ligation, tubal)
Ligne - (Streak; line)
l'immunité - (immunity)
Linéal - (Linear)
Linge - (Clothing)
Lipide - (Lipid)
Lipome - (Lipoma)
Liposoluble - (Liposoluble)
Liqueur - (Liquor)
Liquide - (Liquid)
Liquide amniotique - (Amniotic fluid)

Liquide cérébro-spinal - (Cerebrospinal fluid)
Liquide séminal, sperme - (Semen)
Lisse - (Smooth)
Lit - (Bed)
Lithiase - (Lithiasis)
Lithiase rénale - (Nephrolithiasis)
Lithique - (Lithic; stones, pertaining to)
Litre - (Liter)
Livide - (Pale; livid)
Lividité - (Pallor)
Lobule - (Lobule; lobe)
Local - (Local)
Localisation - (Localization)
Localisé - (Localized)
Lochies - (Lochia)
Locomotion - (Locomotion)
Loger un corps étranger - (Lodge a foreign body, to)
Lombaire - (Lumbar)
Long - (Long)
Longévité - (Longevity)
Longueur - (Length)
Lordose - (Lordosis)
Lotion - (Lotion)
Loucher, strabisme - (Strabismus; crossed eyes)
Lourd (e - (Heavy)
l'oxygène - (oxygen)

Lubrifiant - (Lubricant)
Lumbago - (Lumbago)
Lumière - (Light)
Lunettes - (Glasses;
eyeglasses)
Lunettes - (Glasses;
eyeglasses)
Lunettes bifocales -
(Bifocals)
Lupus - (Lupus)
Luxation - (Dislocation)
luzerne - (alfalfa)
Lymphadénopathie -
(Lymphadenopathy)
Lymphangite -
(Lymphadenitis)
Lymphangite -
(Lymphangitis)
Lymphocyte - (Lymphocyte)
Lymphocytopénie -
(Lymphocytopenia)
Lymphocytose -
(Lymphocytosis)
Lymphome - (Lymphoma)

~ M ~

Macération - (Maceration)
Mâchoire - (Jaw; jawbone)
Mâchoire - (Mandible; jaw)
Macrocéphalie -
(Macrocephaly)

Macrocyte - (Macrocyte)
Macroglossie -
(Macroglossia)
Macrolide - (Macrolide)
Macrophage - (Macrophage)
Maculopapulaire -
(Maculopapular)
Maigrir - (Lose weight;
become thin)
Main - (Hand)
Main droite - (Right hand)
Main gauche - (Left hand)
Maintenant - (Now)
Mais - (But)
Maître / Maîtresse -
(Teacher)
Mal - (Bad)
Mal - (Damage; injury)
Mal a' l'estomac - (Stomach,
sick to the)
Mal aux dents - (Toothache)
Mal aux reins - (Kidney
pain)
Mal de gorge - (Sore throat)
Mal de tête - (Headache)
Mal en point, patraque -
(Chronic illness, person with
a)
Malade - (Sick)
Maladie - (Sickness)
Maladie - (bloat)
maladie - (disease)
maladie aiguë - (acute

disease)
Maladie génétique -
(Genetic disease)
Maladie grave - (Serious
disease)
maladie infectieuse -
(infectious disease)
Maladie
infectieuse,transmissible -
(Infectious disease;
transmissible)
Maladie soudaine - (Sudden
disease)
Maladie terminale -
(Terminal disease)
Maladie vénérienne -
(Venereal disease)
maladies chroniques -
(chronic disease)
Maladies sexuellement
transmissibles MST -
(Sexually Transmitted
Infection; STI)
Maladies transmissibles -
(Transmissible diseases)
Malaire - (Malar; cheek,
relating to the)
Malaire, jugal - (Jugal)
Malaise, douleur - (Malaise)
Malaria - (Malaria)
Malformation -
(Malformation)

Maligne - (Malignant)
Malnutri (e), sous-
alimenté(e - (Malnourished)
Malnutrition - (Malnutrition)
Malnutrition - (Malnutrition)
Maman - (Mother)
Mamelon - (Areola (women)
/ nipple (men); baby
bottle/pacifier)
Mamelon - (Nipple)
Mamelon - (Nipple)
Mammaire - (Mammary)
Mammographie -
(Mammogram;
mammography)
Manchot - (One-handed)
mange maladie - (mange)
Manger - (Eat)
Maniaco-dépressif (ive -
(Manic-depressive)
Manie - (Mania)
Manifestation -
(Manifestation)
Manivelle du sternum -
(Sternal angle;
manubriosternal joint)
Manœuvre - (Maneuver)
Manomètre - (Pressure
gauge)
Manque - (Lack; deficiency)
Manque d' érythrocytes -
(Erythrocytopenia)

Marasme - (Marasmus; wasting)
Marche - (March; progress)
Marcher - (Walk, to)
Marcher, se promener - (Walk, to; to ride)
mari - (Spouse)
Marié(e - (Married)
Marihuana - (Marijuana)
Marque - (Mark; brand)
Marron - (Brown)
Masculin - (Masculine)
Masque - (Mask)
Masque d'oxygène - (Oxygen mask)
Massage - (Massage)
Massage cardiaque - (Cardiac massage)
Masse - (Mass)
Masséter - (Masseter)
Masseur - (Massage therapist; masseur/masseuse)
Mastectomie - (Mastectomy)
Masticateur - (Chewer)
Mastiquer, mâcher - (Chew, to)
Mastite - (Mastitis)
mastite - (mastitis)
Mastocyte - (Mastocyte)
Mastodynie, mastalgie - (Mastodynia; mastalgia)
Mastoïde - (Mastoid)

Mastoïdite - (Mastoiditis)
Matelas - (Mattress)
Maternité - (Maternity)
Matières fécales - (Fecal matter)
Matrice, utérus - (Womb; uterus)
Matrone, femme-sage - (Matron)
Maturation - (Maturation)
Mauvais - (Bad/sick)
Mauvais oeil - (Evil eye)
Mauvais pronostic - (Prognosis, bad)
Mauvaise absorption - (Malabsorption)
Mauvaise absorption intestinale - (Malabsorption, intestinal)
Mauvaise haleine - (Breath, bad)
Maxillaire - (Jaw; maxillary)
Maxillaire inférieur - (Jaw, lower)
Maxillaire supérieur - (Jaw, upper)
Maximal (e - (Maximum)
Maximisation - (Potentiation)
Méat - (Meatus)
Mécanisme - (Mechanism)
Méconium - (Meconium)
Méconnaissance -

(Ignorance; lack of knowledge)
Médecin - (Doctor)
Médecin de famille - (Doctor, family)
Médecin légiste - (Forensic)
Médecine - (Medicine)
Médecine communautaire - (Medicine, community)
Médecine familiale - (Medicine, family)
Médecine préventive - (Medicine, preventative)
Médecine sportive - (Medicine, sport)
Médecine traditionnelle - (Medicine, traditional)
Médiastin - (Mediastinum)
Médicament - (Medicine)
Médicament - (Medicine; remedy(home remedy))
Médicament contra la grippeavec paracétamol - (Anti-flu medication with paracetamol)
Médication - (Medication)
Médicinal - (Medicinal)
Médullaire - (Medullary)
Mégacaryocyte - (Megakaryocyte)
Mégacôlon - (Megacolon)
Méiose - (Meiosis)

Mélange - (Mixture)
Mélanome - (Melanoma)
mélanome - (melanoma)
Méléna - (Melena)
Membrane - (Membrane)
Membrane cellulaire - (Membrane, cellular)
Membre - (Limb; member)
Membre endormi - (Limb asleep e.g.: My leg is asleep)
même - (bile)
Mémoire - (Memory)
Menace - (Threat)
Menarchie - (Menarche)
Méninges - (Meninges)
Méningite - (Meningitis)
Méningo-encéphalite - (Meningoencephalitis)
Ménopause - (Menopause)
Ménopause - (Menopause)
Ménorragie - (Menorrhagia)
Menstruel - (Menstrual)
Mental - (Mental)
Menton - (Chin)
Menton - (Chin, tip of the)
Mère - (Mother)
Mère célibataire - (Mother, single)
Mésentère - (Mesentery)
Mésogastre - (Mesogastrium)

Mesurer - (Measure)
Métabolisme - (Metabolism)
Métabolite - (Metabolite)
Métacarpe - (Metacarpus)
Métaphyse - (Metaphysis)
Métaplasie - (Metaplasia)
Métastase - (Metastasis)
Métastatique - (Metastatic)
Météorisme - (Bloated)
Métrorragie - (Metrorrhagia)
Mettre du plâtre - (Plaster, to put in; cast, to)
Mettre un bandage - (Bandage, to)
Mettre un cathéter, cathétériser - (Catheterize, to)
Micro-bactérie - (Mycobacteria)
Microbe - (Microbe)
microbe - (microbe)
Microbiologie - (Microbiology)
Microorganisme - (Microorganism)
Microscope - (Microscope)
microscope - (microscope)
Microscopique - (Microscopic)
Midi - (Noon)
Mieux, meilleur - (Better than)
Migraine - (Migraine)

Migraine - (Migraine)
Milieu, demi - (Medium; half)
Milligramme - (Milligram)
Mince - (Thin)
minérale - (mineral)
Minéralocorticoïde - (Mineralocorticoid)
Minimal - (Minimal)
Minuit - (Midnight)
Minute - (Minute)
Mise au monde, accoucher - (Birth)
mite - (mite)
Mitose - (Mitosis)
Mitral - (Mitral)
Mobilisation - (Mobilization)
Mobilité - (Mobility)
Modéré (e - (Moderate)
Modification - (Modification)
modifier - (Alter)
modifier - (modify)
Moelle - (Marrow)
Moelle épinière - (Spinal cord)
Moignon - (Stump)
Moitié - (Half)
Molaire - (Molar)
Molaires - (Molars)
Môle - (Mole)
Molécule - (Molecule)
Mollet - (Calf (of leg))
Moment - (Moment)

Moment - (Moment)
Moniteur - (Monitor)
Monitorage - (Monitoring)
Mono-articulaire -
(Monoarticular)
Monocyte - (Monocyte)
Mononucléose infectieuse -
(Mononucleosis, infectious)
Monoplégie - (Monoplegia)
Mono-thérapie -
(Monotherapy)
Montrer - (Teach, to; show,
to)
Morbidité - (Morbidity)
Moribond (e - (Moribund)
Morphine - (Morphine)
Morsure - (Bite)
Mort encéphalique - (Death
encephalic; brain death)
Mort subite - (Death,
sudden; sudden infant
death syndrome)
Mort, cadavre - (Dead;
cadaver)
Mort, décès - (Death)
Mortalité - (Mortality)
Mortalité infantile -
(Mortality, infant)
Mortalité maternelle -
(Mortality, maternal)
Mortel - (Lethal)
Mortel - (Mortal)

Morve, crotte de nez -
(Mucus; snot)
Moteur - (Motor)
Motilité - (Motility)
Motilité intestinale -
(Motility, intestinal)
Motivation - (Motivation)
Mou/Molle - (Soft; bland)
Mouche - (Fly)
Mouillé (e - (Wet; damp)
Mourant(e - (Dying person)
Mourir - (Die, to)
Mourir, décéder - (Die, to;
pass away, to)
Moustique - (Mosquito)
Mouvement - (Movement)
Mucocutané -
(Mucocutaneous)
Mucolytique - (Mucolytic)
mucus - (mucus)
Muet - (Mute)
Multi-factoriel -
(Multifactorial)
Multi-focal - (Multifocal)
Multipare - (Multipara)
Multiple - (Multiple)
Muqueuse - (Mucous)
muqueuse - (mucous
membrane)
Mur - (Wall)
Murmure - (Murmur)
Murmure cardiaque -

(Murmur, heart; cardiac murmur)
Murmure respiratoire, murmure vésiculaire - (Murmur respiratory; vesicular breath sounds)
Murmure systolique - (Murmur, systolic)
Muscle - (Muscle)
Muscle lisse - (Muscle, smooth)
Muscle-squelettique - (Musculoskeletal)
Musculaire - (Muscular)
musculaires - (muscle)
Musculature - (Musculature)
Mutation - (Mutation)
Mutisme - (Mutism)
Myalgie - (Myalgia)
Myasthénie - (Myasthenia)
mycoplasmav microbes semblables à des bactéries (p. 88). - (mycoplasmav Microbes similar to bacteria .)
Mycosis - (Mycosis)
Mycotique - (Mycotic)
Mydriase - (Mydriasis)
Mydriatique - (Mydriatic)
Myéline - (Myelin)
Myélite - (Myelitis)
Myélographie - (Myelography)

Myélome - (Myeloma)
Myeloméningocèles - (Myelomeningocele (MMC))
myiasis - (myiasis)
Myocarde - (Myocardium)
Myocardite - (Myocarditis)
Myologie - (Myology)
Myome - (Myoma)
Myopathie - (Myopathia)
Myopie - (Myopia)
Myosis - (Myosis)
Myotique - (Myotic)
Myxœdème - (Myxedema)
Myxomatose - (Myxomatosis)

~ N ~

Nævus - (Birthmark; mole)
Naissance - (Birth)
Naissance prématurée - (Birth, premature)
Naître - (Born, to be)
Narcotique - (Narcotic)
Natalité - (Birth rate)
Nausées - (Nauseous)
navire - (vessel)
Nébulisation - (Nebulization)
Nébuliseur - (Nebulizer)
Nécropsie - (Autopsy)
Nécrose - (Necrosis)
Négatif (ive - (Negative)

Négation - (Refusal)
Négatoscope - (Negatoscope)
Négligence médicale - (Negligence, medical)
Némathelminthe - (Nemathelminthe)
Nématode - (Nematode)
nématodes - (nematodes)
Néonatal - (Neonatal)
Néoplasie - (Tumor)
Néoplasique - (Neoplastic)
Néphrectomie - (Nephrectomy)
Néphrétique - (Nephritic)
Néphrite - (Nephritis)
Néphrologie - (Nephrology)
Néphropathie - (Nephropathy)
Néphrose - (Nephrosis)
Néphrotoxique - (Nephrotoxic)
Nerf - (Nerve)
nerfs - (nerves)
Nerveux - (Nervous)
Nervosité - (Nervousness)
Neural - (Neural)
Neurasthénie - (Nervous exhaustion)
Neurobiologie - (Neurobiology)
Neurochirurgie -

(Neurosurgery)
Neurochirurgien - (Neurosurgeon)
Neuroleptique - (Neuroleptic)
Neurologie - (Neurology)
Neurologue - (Neurologist)
Neuromusculaire - (Neuromuscular)
Neurone - (Neuron)
Neuropathie - (Neuropathy)
Neuropathologie - (Neuropathology)
Neuropsychiatrie - (Neuropsychiatry)
Neurotoxique - (Neurotoxic)
Neurotropisme - (Neurotropism)
Neutralisation - (Neutralization)
Neutropénie - (Neutropenia)
Neutrophilie - (Neutrophilia)
Neuvième - (Ninth)
Névralgie - (Neuralgia)
Névrite - (Neuritis)
Névrose - (Neurosis)
Névrotique - (Neurotic)
Nez - (Nose)
Niacinamide - (Niacine)
Nicotine - (Nicotine)
Nicotinique - (Nicotinic)
Nistatine - (Nystatin)

Nitroglycérine - (Nitroglycerine)

Niveau - (Level; standard)

Niveaux d´attention de santé - (Health standards)

Nocif - (Harmful)

Nodulaire - (Nodular)

Nodule - (Nodule)

Nœud - (Knot)

Noir, noire - (Black)

Nom - (Name)

Nom de famille - (Last name)

Nombril - (Belly button)

nombril - (navel)

non coordonnée - (uncoordinated)

Non nécessaire - (Unnecessary)

Non- respect - (Non-compliance; non-fulfillment)

Non spécifique - (Unspecific)

Noradrénaline - (Noradrenaline)

Normal - (Normal)

Normalisation - (Normalization)

Nosographie - (Nosography)

Nosologie - (Nosology)

Nostalgie - (Nostalgia)

Notalgie - (Notalgia)

Noter - (Note, to)

Notification - (Notification)

Nourrice - (Nurse, wet)

Nourrir - (Nourish, to; feed, to)

Nourrisson - (Nursing infant)

Nourriture - (Food)

Nourriture saine - (Healthy food)

Nouveau-né - (Newborn)

Nouveau-né (e - (Newborn)

Novocaïne - (Novocaine)

Noyau - (Nucleus)

Nuisible - (Prejudicial; harmful)

Nuit - (Night)

Nul(le - (Null)

Nullipare - (Nullipara)

Numéro - (Number)

Nuque - (Neck, nape of the)

Nutriment - (Nutrient)

Nutritif (ive - (Nutritious)

Nutrition - (Nutrition)

Nycturie - (Nicturia)

nymphe - (nymph)

Nymphomanie - (Nymphomania)

Nystagmus - (Nystagmus)

~ O ~

Obèse - (Obese)

Obésité - (Obesity)
Objectif - (Objective)
Oblitération - (Obliteration)
Observation - (Observation)
Observer - (Observe, to)
Obsession - (Obsession)
Obsolète - (Obsolete)
Obstétricien - (Obstetrician)
Obstétrique - (Obstetrics)
Obstruction - (Obstruction)
Obturer - (Seal, to)
Obtus - (Obtuse)
Occasionnel - (Occasional)
Occasionner - (Cause, to)
Occipital - (Occipital)
Occlure - (Occlude)
Occlusion - (Occlusion, to cause)
Oculaire - (Ocular)
ocytocine - (oxytocin)
Odeur - (Odor)
Odinophagie - (Odyphagia)
Odontalgie - (Toothache)
Odontoblastome - (Odontoblastoma)
Odontocèles - (Odontocele)
Odontologie - (Odontology)
Odontologie préventive - (Dental care, preventive)
Odontologiste - (Odontologist)
Odontome - (Odontoma)

Odontophobie - (Odontophobia)
Odorat - (Smell, sense of)
Oedémateux (euse - (Edematous)
Oedème - (Edema)
Oeil, yeux(pl - (Eye)
Oesophage - (Esophagus)
oesophage - (oesophagus)
oestrus - (oestrus)
Oeuf - (Egg)
Office Panaméricain de la Santé - (Pan-American Health Organization)
Oignon - (Bunion)
Oligomenorrhée - (Oligomenorrhea)
Oligophrène - (Retarded, mentally)
Oligophrénie - (Retardation, mental)
Oligurie - (Oliguria)
omasum - (omasum)
Ombilical - (Umbilical)
Omoplate - (Scapula)
Omphalite - (Omphalitis)
Oncle - (Uncle)
Oncologie, cancérologie - (Oncology)
Oncotique - (Oncotic)
Onde - (Wave)
Ongle - (Nail)

Onguent - (Ointment)
Opacité - (Opacity)
Opérable - (Operable)
Opération - (Operation)
Opération de sauvetage - (Search and rescue)
Opération risquée - (Operation, risky)
Opérer - (Operate, to)
Ophtalmie - (Ophthalmia)
Ophtalmique - (Ophthalmic)
Ophtalmologique - (Ophthalmologic)
Ophtalmologue - (Ophthalmologist)
Ophtalmologue - (Ophthalmologist)
Ophtalmoscope - (Ophthalmoscope)
Ophtalmoscopie - (Ophthalmoscopy)
Opiacé - (Opiate)
Opiner - (Opinion, to give an)
Opisthotonos - (Opisthotonos)
Opportuniste - (Opportunist)
Opportunité - (Opportunity)
Oppressif (ive - (Oppress)
Oppression - (Oppression)
Opthalmologie - (Ophthalmology)

Optimal - (Optimum)
Optique - (Optical)
Optométriste - (Optometrist)
Oral - (Oral)
Orbitaire, orbital - (Orbital)
Orbite - (Orbit)
Orchite - (Orchitis)
Ordinateur - (Computer)
Ordonnance - (Prescription)
Ordonnance, recette - (Prescription)
Ordures, déchets, résidus - (Trash)
Oreille - (Ear)
Oreille - (Ear (outer))
Oreillon - (Mumps)
Organe - (Organ)
Organe ajouté (e, es - (Adjacent organ)
Organe ajouté (e, es - (Adnexa)
Organes de l'œil :sourcils, cils, paupières, glandes lacrymales. - (Eye adnexa)
Organisation Mondiale de laSanté - (World Health Organization)
Organisme - (Organism)
organisme - (organism)
Orgasme - (Orgasm)
Orgelet - (Stye)
Orientation - (Orientation)

Orifice - (Orifice)
Origine - (Origin)
Oropharynx - (Oropharynx)
Orteils - (Toes)
Orthodontie -
(Orthodontics)
Orthopédique - (Orthopedic)
Orthopnée - (Orthopnea)
Orthostatique - (Orthostatic)
Os - (Bone)
Os cassé - (Fracture,
hairline)
Os du nez - (Septum, Nasal)
Os scapulaire - (Scapula;
shoulder blade)
Osmotique - (Osmotic)
Osseux (se - (Bone)
Ossification - (Ossification)
Ostéalgie - (Ostealgia)
Ostéite - (Osteitis)
Ostéo-arthrite -
(Osteoarthritis)
Ostéo-arthrose -
(Osteoarthrosis)
Ostéochondrose -
(Osteocondritis)
Ostéo-dystrophie -
(Osteodystrophy)
Ostéolyse - (Osteolysis)
Ostéomalacie -
(Ostemalacia)
Ostéomyélite -

(Osteomyelitis)
Ostéopathie - (Osteopathy)
Ostéophyte - (Osteophyte)
Ostéoplastie - (Osteoplasty)
Ostéoporose -
(Osteoporosis)
Ostéosarcome -
(Osteosarcoma)
Otalgie - (Earache)
Otite - (Otitis)
Oto- rhino- laryngologie -
(Ear nose & throat, Study
of; ENT)
Otolaryngologie - (Ear and
throat, study of)
Otologie - (Otology)
Oto-mycose - (Otomycosis)
Otorragie - (Otorrhagia)
Otorrhée - (Otorrhea)
Otosclérose - (Otosclerosis)
Otoscope - (Otoscope)
Oto-toxique - (Ototoxic)
Ouvert - (Open)
Ouverture - (Opening)
Ouvrir - (Open, to)
Ouvrir, découvrir -
(Uncover)
Ovaire - (Ovary)
ovaire - (ovary)
Ovule - (Ovule; ovum; egg)
Ovuler - (Ovulate)
Oxygénation -

(Oxygenation)
Oxygène - (Oxygen)
Oxygénothérapie -
(Oxigenotherapy)
Oxymétrie - (Oxymetry)
Oxytocine - (Oxytocin)

~ P ~

Pacemaker, stimulateur
cardiaque - (Pacemaker)
Pain - (Bread)
Palais - (Palate)
Pâle - (Pale)
Pâleur - (Pallor)
Pâlir - (Pale, to become)
Palliatif (ive - (Palliative)
Palpable - (Palpable)
Palpation - (Palpation)
Palpébral - (Palpebral)
Palpitation - (Palpitation)
Paludisme - (Malaria)
Panacée - (Panacea)
Panaris - (Whitlow; pale and
sickly person)
Pancréas - (Pancreas)
Pancréatite - (Pancreatitis)
Pancytopénie -
(Pancytopenia)
Panniculite - (Panniculitis)
Pansement - (Dressing)
Pansement adhésif - (Band-

aid)
Pantalon - (Trousers; pants)
Papa - (Father; dad; papa)
Papier - (Paper; role)
Papillœdème -
(Papilledema)
Papule, nodule - (Papule)
Paracentèse - (Paracentesis)
Para-influenza -
(Parainfluenza)
Parallèle - (Parallel)
Paralyse - (Paralysis)
Paralysé des deux côtés -
(Diplagia)
Paralyser - (Paralyze)
Paralytique - (Paralytic)
paralytique - (Paralyzed)
Paramédical - (Paramedic;
paramedical)
Paramètres - (Parameter)
Paranoïa - (Paranoia)
Paraphimosis -
(Paraphimosis)
Paraplégie - (Paraplegia)
Paraplégique - (Paraplegic)
Parasitaire - (Parasitic)
parasitaire gastro-entérite -
(parasitic gastro-enteritis)
parasite - (parasite)
Parasité (e - (Parasitized)
Parasites - (Parasites)
Parasitisme - (Parasitism)
Parasternal - (Parasternal)

Parasympathique - (Parasympathetic)
Parathyroïdes - (Parathyroid)
Parenchyme - (Parenchyma)
Parentéral - (Parenteral)
Parents - (Progenitor; parent)
Parents - (Relative, a)
Parésie - (Paresis)
Parétique - (Paretic)
Parkinsonismes, variations dumal de Parkinson - (Parkinsonism)
Parler - (Speak, to)
Paronichie - (Paronychia)
Parotide - (Parotid)
Parotidite, oreillon - (Parotiditis (mumps))
Paroxysmale - (Paroxysmal)
Partenaire - (Partner)
Particule - (Particle)
Partie - (Genitalia, female)
Partie arrière - (Back of, the; behind, the)
Passage, billet - (Passage)
Passé - (Past)
Pastille - (Pill)
Pâte - (Paste (noun))
Pathogène - (Pathogenic)
Pathogénie - (Pathogen)
Pathognomonique - (Pathognomonic)
Pathologique - (Pathologic)
Patient - (Patient)
Patte - (Foot; paw)
Paume - (Palm)
Paume de la main - (Palm of the hand)
Paupière - (Eyelid)
Pause - (Pause)
Pauvre - (Poor)
Pauvreté - (Poverty)
Pavillon de l'oreille - (Auricle (of external ear))
Peau - (Skin)
Peau - (Skin)
Peau (couleur - (Complexion)
peau conjonctive - (conjunctiva)
Peau de visage - (Complexion; skin)
Peau gercée - (Skin, cracked)
Pectoral - (Pectoral)
Pédiatre - (Pediatrician)
Pédiatrie - (Pediatrics)
Pédiatrique - (Pediatric)
Pédiculose - (Pediculosis)
Pellagre - (Pellagra)
Pelvien - (Pelvic)
Pénicilline - (Penicillin)
Pénis - (Penis)

pénis - (penis)
Pénis, priape - (Penis)
Penser - (Think, to)
Peptique - (Peptic)
Perception - (Perception)
Percussion - (Percussion)
Percutané (e - (Percutaneous)
Percuter - (Percuss, to; to strike)
Perdre - (Lose, to)
Perdre du sang - (Lose blood, to)
Père - (Father)
Perforation - (Perforation)
Perfusion - (Perfusion)
Péri-anal - (Perianal)
Périarthrite - (Periarthritis)
Péricarde - (Pericardium)
Péricardite - (Pericarditis)
Périnatal - (Perinatal)
Périnéal - (Perineal)
Périnée - (Perineum)
Période - (Period; menstruation)
Période de repos - (Rest period)
Périodique - (Periodic; newspaper or magazine)
Péristaltique - (Peristalltic)
Péritoine - (Peritoneum)
Péritonéal - (Peritoneal)
Péritonite - (Peritonitis)

Perméable - (Permeable; not water proof)
Permis - (Permission)
Pernicieux - (Pernicious)
Péroné - (Fibula)
Persistant - (Persistent)
Personnalité - (Personality)
Personne âgée - (Senior citizen)
Personne saine - (Healthy person)
Personnel de la santé - (Health personnel)
Perte de conscience - (Dizziness)
Perte de la connaissance - (Loss of consciousness)
Perte de la voix - (Loss of voice)
Perversion - (Perversion)
Pétéchie - (Petechia)
Petit (e - (Small)
Petit fils/ Petite fille - (Grandchild)
Peu - (Little)
Peur - (Fear)
Phagocytaire - (Phagocytic)
Phagocyte - (Phagocyte)
Phagocyter - (Phagocytize)
Phagocytose - (Phagocytosis)
Phalange - (Phalange)
Phallus - (Phallus)

Pharmaceutique - (Pharmaceutical)
Pharmacie - (Drugstore; Pharmacy)
Pharmacie - (Pharmacy; drug store)
Pharmacien - (Phamacist; druggist)
Pharmacocinétique - (Pharmacokinetic)
Pharmacodépendance - (Prescription drug dependency)
Pharmacodynamie - (Pharmacodynamics)
Pharmacodynamique - (Pharmacodynamic)
Pharmacologie - (Pharmacology)
Pharmacologue - (Pharmacologist)
Pharmacopée - (Pharmacopoeia)
Pharyngé (e - (Pharyngeal)
Pharyngite - (Pharyngitis)
Pharyngo-amydalite - (Pharyngotonsillitis)
Pharyngo-laryngite - (Pharyngolaryngitis)
Pharyngoscope - (Pharyngoscope)
Pharyngoscopie -

(Pharyngoscopy)
Pharyngotomie - (Pharyngotomy)
Pharynx - (Pharynx)
Phase - (Phase)
Phénobarbital - (Phenobarbitol)
Phénomène - (Phenomenon)
Phénotype - (Phenotype)
Phéochromocytome - (Pheochromocytoma)
Phimosis - (Phimosis)
Phlébite - (Phlebitis)
Phléborragie - (Phleborrhagia)
Phlébothrombose - (Phlebothrombosis)
Phlébotomie - (Phlebotomy)
Phlegmon, abcès dentaire - (Phlegmon, dental abcess)
Phobie - (Phobia)
Phocomélie - (Phocomelia)
Phosphate - (Phosphate)
Phosphaturie - (Phosphaturia)
Phosphorisme - (Phosphorism)
Photophobie - (Photophobia)
Photophobie - (Photophobia)

Photosensibilité - (Photosensitivity)
Photosensible - (Photosensitive)
Photothérapie - (Phototherapy)
Phrénique - (Phrenic)
Phtisique, tuberculeux - (Consumptive)
Physiologie - (Physiology)
Physiologique - (Physiologic; physiological)
Physionomie - (Appearance; features)
Physiopathologie - (Pathophysiology)
Physiothérapeute - (Physical therapist)
Physiothérapie - (Physical therapy)
Physique - (Physical; physique)
Picotement, démangeaison - (Pruritus)
Pied - (Foot, human)
Pieds nus - (Barefoot)
Pierre, caillou - (Stone)
Pierres aux reins - (Stones, kidney; renal calculi)
Pigmentation - (Pigmentation)
Piloérection - (Piloerection)
Pilule - (Pill (specifically a contraceptive pill))
Pince - (Tweezers; forceps; clamps)
pinces - (pliers)
Piquer - (Itch, to)
Piquer - (Pierce, to; to puncture; to prick)
Piqûre - (Bite (e.g. of insect))
Piqûre de moustique - (Bite, mosquito)
Pire - (Worse)
Piston - (Embolus, emboli (pl))
Pityriasis - (Pityriasis)
Placebo - (Placebo)
Placenta - (Placenta)
placenta - (placenta)
Placer, mettre - (Put, to)
Plaie - (Ulcer; sore)
Plainte - (Complaint)
Plainte - (Groan; moan)
Plan, plat - (Plan; flat)
Planification de la santé - (Planning, health)
Planification familiale - (Planning, family; contraception)
Plante - (Plant)
Plante du pied - (Sole; bottom of the foot)
plantes légumineuses - (legume)

Plaquette - (Platelet)
Plasma - (Plasma)
Plâtre - (Plaster)
Plein (e - (Full)
Plénitude - (Plenitude;
abundance)
Pleurer - (Cry, to)
Pleurite - (Pleuritis)
Plèvre - (Pleura)
Plexus - (Plexus)
Pli - (Fold (noun))
Plomb - (Lead (noun))
Plombage - (Filling)
Plus - (More)
Plus grand - (Bigger)
Plus grand que, majeur -
(More than)
Plus petit que, mineur -
(Minor; smaller or less than)
Plusieurs - (Various;
several)
Pneumocoque -
(Pneumococcus)
Pneumocystose -
(Pneumocystis jiroveci)
Pneumonie - (Pneumonia)
Pneumonie - (Pneumonia)
pneumonie - (pneumonia)
Pneumopathie -
(Pneumopathy)
Pneumorragie -
(Pneumorrhagia)

Pneumothorax -
(Pneumothorax)
Poche lacrymale - (Lacrimal
sac)
Poids - (Weight)
Poids à la naissance -
(Weight, birth)
Poids corporel - (Weight,
body)
Poignet - (Fist)
Poignet - (Wrist)
Poil, cheveu - (Hair)
Point - (Point; stitch;
suture)
Pointe - (Point; tip)
Pointillé - (Dotted; stippled;
sutured)
Poire a' lavement - (Enema)
Poison - (Poison)
Poitrine - (Chest)
Poliomyélite - (Poliomyelitis)
Pollen - (Pollen)
Polyarthrite - (Polyarthritis)
Polyclinique - (Polyclinic)
Polycythémie -
(Polycythemia)
Polydipsie - (Polydipsia)
Polygamie - (Polygamy)
Polyhydramnios -
(Polyhydramnios)
Polymorphique -
(Polymorphic)

Polype - (Polyp)
Polyphagie - (Polyphagia)
Polysaccharide - (Polysaccharide)
Polyurie - (Polyuria)
Pommade - (Balsamic)
Pommade - (Ointment)
Pompe - (Pump)
Pomper - (Pump, to)
Ponction - (Puncture)
Ponction lombaire - (Puncture lumbar)
Poplité - (Popliteal)
Population - (Population)
Porte d'entrée - (Entrance; entryway)
Porte de sortie - (Exit)
Porteur - (Carrier)
Poser une question - (Question, to (ask a))
Positif (ive - (Positive)
Position - (Position)
Posologie - (Sig (dosing plan, as in prescription))
Possible - (Possible)
Postérieur - (Posterior)
Post-ménopausique - (Postmenopausal)
Postopératoire - (Postoperative)
Postprandial - (Postprandial)
Posture - (Posture)
Pot de nuit - (Urinal)

Potable - (Potable)
Potion - (Potion)
Potion - (Potion)
Pou - (Flea)
Poubelle - (Trashcan)
Pouce - (Thumb)
Pouce - (Thumb)
Poudre - (Talc)
Poudre, poussière - (Powder; dust)
Pouls - (Pulse)
Poumon - (Lung)
Pour - (For)
Pourpre - (Purpura; purple)
Pourri(e - (Rotten)
Poursuivre - (Continue)
Pousser - (Push, to)
Pouvoir - (Able, to be)
Prandial - (Prandial)
Pré- éclampsie - (Pre-eclampsia)
Préalable - (Previous (or previa, after placenta))
Pré-anesthésie - (Preanesthesia)
Précaire - (Precarious)
Précancéreux - (Precancerous)
Précipitation - (Precipitation)
Pré-clinique - (Preclinical)
Précurseur - (Precursor)
Pré-diabète - (Prediabetic)

Prédisposition - (Predisposition)
Prélèvement d'exsude ou sécrétion suintant - (Exuded)
Préliminaire - (Preliminary)
Prématuré - (Premature)
Prémenstruel - (Premenstrual)
Premier soins - (First aid)
Premier, première - (First)
Première dose, dose initiale - (Initial dose)
Premiers signes d'une épidémie - (Disease outbreak)
Prénatal - (Prenatal)
Préparé (e - (Prepared)
Prépuce - (Prepuce)
Près - (Near; Fence; Hedge)
Prescription facultative - (Doctor's orders)
Prescription médicale - (Prescription, medical)
Prescrire - (Prescribe)
Prescrire - (Prescribe, to)
Présent - (Present)
Présentation de siège - (Delivery; breech)
Préservatif - (Condom)
Pression sanguine systolique - (Pressure, systolic blood)

Pression, tension - (Pressure)
Pression, tension osmotique - (Pressure, osmotic)
Prévalence - (Prevalence)
Prévenir - (Prevent, to)
Prévention - (Prevention)
Prévention de santé - (Prevention, health)
Priapisme - (Priapism)
Primaire - (Primary)
Primipare - (Primipara)
Primitif - (Primitive)
Principal - (Principal)
Printemps - (Spring (the season))
Prioritaire - (Priority)
Privation - (Privation; deprivation; loss)
Privation d'aliment pendantlongtemps - (Inanition; fasting)
Prix - (Price)
Probabilité - (Probability)
Problème - (Problem)
Procédure - (Procedure)
Processus - (Process (in some sites may mean medical chart))
Prochain (e - (Next to)
Proche - (Nearby)
Proctalgie - (Proctalgia)

Proctite, rectite - (Proctitis)
Proctocèles - (Rectocele)
Prodrome - (Prodrome)
Produit - (Product)
Produit médicinal - (Medicinal product)
Profession - (Profession)
Professionnel (le - (Professional)
Profondeur - (Depth)
Progestérone - (Progesterone)
Programme de santé - (Program, health)
Progrès médical - (Medical advance)
Progressif (ive - (Progressive)
Prohibition d'aliments - (NPO; fasting)
Prolapsus - (Prolapse)
Prolifération - (Proliferation)
Prolongé (e - (Prolonged)
Promiscuité - (Promiscuity)
Promotion de santé - (Promotion, health)
Prompt - (Soon)
Pronostic - (Prognosis)
Pronostiquer - (Prognosticate)
Propanolol - (Propranolol)
Propédeutique - (Preparatory studies)

Prophylaxie - (Prophylaxis)
Propre - (Clean)
Propre - (Own (as in his own, her own) or to be correct; appropriate)
Prospectus - (Prospectus)
Prostate - (Prostate)
Prostatique - (Prostatic)
Prostatisme - (Prostatism)
Prostatite - (Prostatitis)
Prostration - (Prostration)
Protection radiologique - (Radiologic protection)
Protéger - (Protect, to)
protéin - (protein)
Protéine - (Protein)
Protéines de la diète - (Proteins, dietary)
Protéinurie - (Proteinuria)
Protéolytique - (Proteolytic)
Prothèse - (Prosthesis)
Protoplasme - (Protoplasm)
Protozoaire - (Protozoan)
protozoaires - (protozoa)
Protrusion - (Protrusion)
Protubérance - (Excrescence; protuberance)
Prouver, essayer - (Try, to; try out, to; prove, to)
Proximal - (Proximal)
Prurit - (Pruritus)
Pseudo grossesse -

(Pseudopregnancy)
Pseudo tumeur -
(Pseudotumor)
Psoas - (Psoas)
Psoriasis - (Psoriasis)
Psoriasis - (Psoriasis)
Psychiatre - (Psychiatrist)
Psychiatrie - (Psychiatry)
Psychiatrique - (Psychiatric)
Psychiatrique - (Psychiatrist)
Psychologique -
(Psychological)
Psychomoteur -
(Psychomotor)
Psychopathe - (Psychopath)
Psychose - (Psychosis)
Psychose - (Psychosis)
Psychosocial -
(Psychosocial)
Psychosomatique -
(Psychosomatic)
Psychothérapie -
(Psychotherapy)
Psychotrope - (Medication,
psychiatric)
Ptérygion - (Pterygium)
Ptôsis, ptôse - (Ptosis)
Puberté - (Puberty)
Pubis - (Pubis)
Puer, odeur fétide - (Stink;
foul odor)
Puerpéral, (e, aux -

(Puerperal)
Puissance - (Strength;
potency)
Puits artésien - (Well
(noun), artesian)
Pulmonaire - (Pulmonary)
Pulpe - (Pulp; soft tissue)
Pulsation - (Pulsation)
Pultacé(e - (Macerated)
Pupe - (Pupa)
Pupille - (Pupil)
Pupille - (Pupil (of the eye))
Purée - (Puree)
Purgatif (ve - (Laxative)
Purifier - (Purify, to)
Purpura trombotique
trombocitopénique -
(Purpura;
thrombocytopenic)
Purulent(e - (Purulent)
Pus - (Pus)
pus - (pus)
Pustule - (Pustule)
Pustuleux - (Pustulous)
Pyélonéphrite -
(Pyelonephritis)
Pylore - (Pylorus)
Pyodermie - (Pyoderma)
Pyogène - (Pyogenic)
Pyonéphrite - (Pyonephritis)
Pyrexie - (Pyrexia)
Pyridoxine - (Pyridoxine)

Pyrogène - (Pyrogenic)
Pyrosis - (Pyrosis)
Pyurie - (Pyuria)

~ Q ~

Quadriceps - (Quadriceps)
Quadriplégie -
(Quadriplegia)
Quadriplégique,
tétraplégique -
(Quadriplegic)
Quadruplet - (Quadruplet)
Qualitatif (ve - (Qualitative)
Qualité de l'eau - (Water
quality)
Qualité de vie - (Quality of
life)
Qualité des médicaments -
(Quality of medications)
Quand un cellule meure
acause la membrane est
brisée - (Lysis)
Quantitatif (ve -
(Quantitative)
Quarentaine - (Quarantine)
Question - (Question)
Qui a perdu connaissance -
(Fainted)
Qui a une glycémie normale
- (Normoglycemia)
Qui a une hernie - (Hernia,
having a)
Qui a une température nor-
male - (Normothermia)
Qui a une tension normale -
(Normotensive)
Qui endort - (Sleep
inducing)
Qui souffre d'endocardite -
(Endocarditis)
Quinine - (Quinine)
Quinte de toux - (Coughing
spell)

~ R ~

Race - (Race)
Rachialgie - (Rachialgia)
Rachidien - (Rachidian)
Rachis - (Rachis; spinal
column)
Rachitique - (Rachitic;
rickety)
Rachitisme - (Rickets;
rachitis)
Racial - (Racial)
Racine - (Root)
Radial(le - (Radial)
Radiant (e - (Radiant)
Radiation - (Radiation)
Radical (e - (Radical)
Radiculite - (Radiculitis)
Radio transparent -

(Radiotransparent)
Radiographie - (Radiograph; X-ray)
Radiographie du larynx - (Laryngography)
Radiologie - (Radiology)
Radiologue - (Radiologist)
Radiopaque - (Radiopaque)
Radiothérapie - (Radiation therapy)
Rage - (Rabies; rage)
Raison - (Reason)
Ramollir - (Soften, to)
Ranule, grenouillette - (Ranula)
Râpé - (Curettage; scrape; scraped)
Raphé - (Raphe)
Rapide, vite - (Rapid; fast)
Raréfaction - (Rarefaction)
Rash, éruption cutanée - (Rash, cutaneous eruption)
Rate - (Spleen)
rate - (spleen)
Ration - (Ration; serving)
Rationnel (le - (Rational)
Rauque, enroué (e - (Hoarse)
Rayon X - (X-rays)
Réabsorber - (Reabsorb)
Réabsorption - (Reabsorption)

Réactif - (Reactive)
Réaction - (Reaction)
Réaction adverse à un médicament, RAM - (Adverse drug reaction, ADR)
Réactivation - (Reactivation)
Réactivité - (Reactivity)
Réanimation - (Resuscitation)
Réanimer - (Resuscitate, to)
Recensement - (Census; count)
Récent - (Recent)
Récepteur - (Receptor)
Récessif - (Recessive)
Récession - (Recession)
Recherche, investigation - (Investigation; research)
Rechute - (Relapse)
Récidive - (Recurrence; relapse)
Recommandable - (Recommendable)
Recommandation - (Recommendation)
Recomptage de cellules - (Cell count)
Reconstitution - (Reconstitution)
Record, registre - (Record; file)

Recouvrir la santé -
(Recovery of health)
Rectal - (Rectal)
Rectification - (Rectification;
correction)
Recto sigmoïde -
(Rectosigmoid)
Rectoscopie - (Proctoscopy)
Rectum - (Rectum)
rectum - (rectum)
Récupération -
(Recuperation)
Récurrent - (Recurrent)
Réduction - (Reduction)
Référé (e - (Referred)
Référence - (Reference)
Référer - (Refer, to)
Réflection - (Reflection)
Réflexe - (Reflex)
Réflexe de décortiquement -
(Reflex; decortication)
Reflux - (Reflux)
Reflux gastro-œsophagien -
(Reflux gastroesophageal)
Réfractaire - (Refractory)
Réfractaire a' certaines
maladies - (Immune)
Réfraction - (Refraction)
Refroidissement - (Cooling)
Refus - (Rejection)
Régénération -
(Regeneration)
Régime - (Regimen)

Régime d'amaigrissement -
(Regimen, weight loss)
Régime thérapeutique -
(Regimen, therapeutic)
Région - (Region; area)
Région précordiale -
(Precordial)
Régional - (Regional)
Registre médicale -
(Registry, medical)
Règle - (Menstrual period;
rule; ruler)
Règles, menstruation -
(Menstruation)
Régression - (Regression)
Régulation - (Regulation)
Régulièrement - (Regularly)
Régurgitation -
(Regurgitation)
Réhabilitation -
(Rehabilitation)
Réhydratation -
(Rehydration)
Réhydrater - (Rehydrate, to)
Rein - (Kidney)
Reinfection - (Reinfection)
Relatif à l'aura - (Aural)
Relatif aux neurones -
(Neuronal)
Relatif aux trompes de
Fallopeet l'ovaire -
(Tuboovarian)
Relation - (Relation;

relationship)
Relaxant (e - (Relaxant)
Relaxer - (Relax, to)
Religion - (Religion)
Remède - (Remedy; cure)
Remédier - (Remedy, to; cure, to)
Rémission - (Remission)
Remplacer - (Replace, to)
Remuer - (Remove, to)
Rénal - (Renal)
Réparation d'une valvule cardiaque - (Valvuloplasty)
Repas - (Supper)
Répéter - (Repeat, to)
Réplique - (Reply; copy)
Réponse - (Response; answer)
Reporter - (Report, to)
Repos - (Rest)
Repos - (Rest, a)
Repos au lit - (Rest bed)
Reposer - (Rest, to)
Reposition - (Replacement)
repousser - (repel)
Répression - (Repression)
Reproduction - (Reproduction)
Réseau - (Net; network)
Résection - (Resection)
Réservoir - (Reservoir)
Résiduel (le - (Residual)

Résine - (Resin)
Résistance - (Resistance)
Résistance aux antibiotiques - (Resistance, antibiotic)
Résistance aux médicaments - (Resistance, medication)
résistant - (resistant)
Résistant (e - (Resistant)
Résonance - (Resonance)
Respiration - (Respiration)
Respiration profonde - (Deep breath)
Respiratoire - (Respiratory)
Respirer - (Breathe, to)
Responsable - (Responsible)
Ressources de santé - (Resources, health)
Ressuscitation - (Resuscitation)
Ressusciter - (Resuscitate, to)
Reste - (Surplus)
Rester au lit - (Bed rest)
Résultat - (Result)
Résumé - (Summary)
Résumer - (Summarize, to)
Rétabli (e - (Recovered)
Retard - (Delay; lag)
Retard - (Delay; retardation)
Retard mental -

(Developmental delay;
mental retardation)
Rétention - (Retention)
Rétention de liquides -
(Retention, Fluid)
réticulum - (reticulum)
Rétine - (Retina)
rétine - (retina)
Rétinopathie - (Retinopathy)
Retirer - (Remove, to)
Retourner - (Return, to)
Rétraction - (Retraction)
Rétro lingual - (Retrolingual)
Retro oculaire -
(Retroocular)
Rétro périnée -
(Retroperitoneal)
Rétroflexion - (Retroflexion)
Rétrograde - (Retrograde)
Rétrospectif (ve -
(Retrospective)
Rêve - (Sleep; dream)
Réversible - (Reversible)
Revêtement - (Lining;
covering)
Revivre - (Revive, to)
Revue - (Review; magazine)
Révulsif (ive - (Revulsive)
Rhabdomyolyse -
(Rhabdomyolysis)
Rhinite - (Rhinitis)
Rhinite allergique - (Rhinitis,
allergic)

Rhinopharynx -
(Nasopharynx)
Rhinorrhée - (Rhinorrhea)
Rhumatisme -
(Rheumatism)
Rhumatisme -
(Rheumatism)
Rhumatoïde - (Rheumatoid)
Riboflavine - (Riboflavin)
rickettsies - (rickettsia)
Rides de la peau - (Wrinkles
of the skin)
Rien - (Nothing)
Rifampicine - (Rifampin)
Rigidité - (Rigidity; stiffness)
Rince bouche, bains de
bouche, collutoire -
(Collutorium)
Rinopharyngite -
(Nasopharyngitis)
Rinopharynx -
(Nasopharynx)
Rire - (Laugh)
Risque - (Risk)
Robe, habit - (Dressed)
Rond (e - (Round)
Rose - (Pink)
Rotation - (Rotation)
Rotule - (Patella; kneecap)
Rouge - (Red)
Rougeole - (Measles)
Rougeole - (Rubella)
Rougeur - (Redness;

flushing)
Rougir - (Turn red, to)
Rugueux - (Rough)
rumen - (rumen)
ruminants - (ruminant)
ruminer - (ruminate)
Rupture - (Rupture)
Rythme - (Rhythm)
Rythme cardiaque - (Rhythm, cardiac)
Rythmique - (Rhythmic)

~ S ~

S'allonger, rallonger, prolonger - (Lengthen, to; longer, to get)
S'enrhumer - (Cold, to catch a)
Sac - (Sac)
Sac de glace - (Ice bag)
Saccharine - (Saccharine)
Saccharose - (Sweet)
Sacro lombaire - (Sacrolumbar)
Sage femme, matrone - (Midwife)
Sagittal - (Sagittal)
Saignée - (Bleeding)
Saignée gastro-intestinale - (Bleeding, Gastrointestinal)

Saignement - (Bleeding; bloody)
Saigner - (Bleed, to)
Saigner - (Bleed, to)
Sain - (Healthy (sound))
Sain (e), en bonne santé - (Healthy)
Saindoux - (Lard)
Sale - (Dirty)
Salé - (Salty)
Salicylate - (Salicylate)
Salicylisme - (Salicylism (salicylate toxicity))
Salive - (Saliva)
salive - (saliva)
Salle d´opération - (Room operating (surgical))
Salle d'accouchement - (Room, delivery)
Salle d'attente - (Room, waiting)
Salle d'opération - (Operating room)
Salle de récupération - (Room, recovery)
Salmonelle - (Salmonella)
Salon d'opération - (Room, operating)
Salpingite - (Salpingitis)
Salubre - (Safe (salubrious))
Saluer - (Greet, to)
Sang - (Blood)

Sang caché - (Blood, Occult)
Sang veineux - (Blood, Venous)
Sanitaire - (Sanitary)
Sans différence - (Undifferentiated)
Sans fièvre - (Afebrile)
Santé - (Health)
Santé buccale - (Health, oral)
Santé de la mère et du nouveau-né - (Health, maternal-child)
Santé environnementale - (Health, environmental)
Santé mentale - (Health, mental)
Santé publique - (Health, public)
Saphène - (Saphenous)
Saprophyte - (Saprophyte)
sarcoïde - (sarcoid)
Sarcome - (Sarcoma)
Sarcome de Kaposi - (Sarcoma, kaposi's)
sarcopte de la gale - (Parasite)
Saturation - (Saturation)
Saturation d'oxygène - (Saturation, oxygen)
Saturnisme - (Poisoning, lead)

Sauter - (Jump, to)
Sauver - (Save, to)
Saveur - (Taste)
Savoir - (Know, to)
Savon - (Soap)
Scabicide - (Scabicide)
Scabiose, gale - (Scabies)
Scalpel, bistouri - (Scalpel)
Scarlatine - (Scarlet fever)
Schizophrénie - (Schizophrenia)
Sciatique - (Sciatica)
Science - (Science)
Sclérose - (Sclerosis)
Sclérotique - (Sclerotic)
Scoliose - (Scoliosis)
Scorbut - (Scurvy)
Scrotum - (Scrotum)
scrotum - (scrotum)
Se communiquer - (Communicate)
Se coucher - (Lie down, to; go to bed, to)
Se gratter - (Scratch oneself, to)
Se lever - (Get up, to; stand, to)
Se noyer, s'étouffer - (Drown, to; choke, to)
Se plaindre - (Groan, to; complain, to)
Se rappeler - (Remember, to)

Se relaxer - (Relax oneself, to)
Se rétablir - (Recover, to)
Séborrhée - (Seborrhea)
Sec, sèche - (Dry)
Sécher - (Dry, to)
Secondaire - (Secondary)
Secourir - (Relieve, to; to aide)
Secrétariat - (Secretary)
Sécrétion - (Secretion)
Sédatif - (Sedative)
Sédentaire - (Sedentary)
Sédiment - (Sediment)
Sédimentation - (Sedimentation)
Segment - (Segment)
Ségrégation - (Segregation)
Sein - (Breast)
Sein - (Sinus; breast)
Sel - (Salt)
Sélectif (ve - (Selective)
Sélection - (Selection)
Sélectionner - (Select, to)
Semaine - (Week)
Sémiotique - (Semiotic)
Sénile - (Senile)
Sénilité - (Senility)
Sens - (Sense (5 senses or instinct))
Sensation - (Sensation)
Sensibilisation - (Sensitization)
Sensibilité - (Sensitivity)
Sensible - (Sensible)
Sensoriel (le - (Sensory)
Sensuel - (Sensual)
Sentiment - (Feeling)
Sentir - (Feel)
Sentir - (Smell, to)
Séparation - (Separation)
Sepsis, infection - (Sepsis)
Septicémie - (Septicemia)
septicémie - (septicaemia)
Septique - (Septic)
Séquelles - (Sequelae)
Sérieux(se - (Serious)
Seringue - (Syringe)
Sérologie - (Serology)
Sérologique - (Serological)
Séronégatif (ive - (Seronegative)
Séropositif (ive - (Seropositive)
Sérotype - (Serotype)
Sérovigilance - (Serovigilance)
Serpent - (Snake)
Sérum - (Serum)
Service d'Urgences - (Emergency medical team)
Service de gynécologie etobstétrique - (Obstetric services; gynecological

services)
Service sanitaire - (Health)
Seul (e - (Alone; only)
Sevrage - (Weaning)
Sevrer - (Wean, to)
sevrer - (wean)
Sexe - (Sex; intercourse)
Sexualité - (Sexuality)
Shigella - (Shigella)
Shigellose - (Shigellosis)
Sialagogue - (Sialogogues)
SIDA - (AIDS)
Sidéropénie - (Siderosis)
Sieste - (Nap)
Sigmoïde - (Sigmoid;
sigmoidal)
Signal - (Signal)
Signature - (Signature)
Signe - (Sign)
Significatif - (Significant)
Similaire - (Similar)
Simulé (e - (Simulated)
Sinus nasaux - (Sinuses
paranasal)
Sinusite - (Sinusitis)
Sirop - (Syrup)
Situation - (Situation)
Sixième - (Sixth)
Société - (Society)
Soif - (Thirst)
Soigner - (Assist)
Soigner - (Care for, to)
Soigner - (Cure, to)

Soin - (Care)
Soin à long terme - (Long-
term care)
Soin ambulatoire -
(Ambulatory care)
Soin de l'enfant -
(Childcare)
Soin du convalescent -
(Care of convalescent)
Soin maternel - (Maternal
care)
Soin pendant
l'allaitement,soin du
nourrison - (Care for
unweaned babies)
Soin post-opératoire - (Post-
operative care)
Soin pour prolonger la vie -
(Care for a prolonged life)
Soin pré-opératoire - (Pre-
operative care)
Soin terminal - (Terminal
care)
Soins d'urgence -
(Emergency care)
Soins d'urgence - (Urgent
Care)
Soins médicaux - (Medical
care)
Soins santé primaire -
(Primary care)
Soins secondaires -
(Secondary care)

Soins tertiaires - (Tertiary care)
Soins, aide - (Help)
Soleil - (Sun)
Solide - (Solid)
Soluble - (Soluble)
Solution - (Solution)
Solution aqueuse - (Aqueous)
Solution pour faire des gargarismes - (Solution, gargling)
Solution saline - (Solution, saline)
Soma - (Soma)
Somatique - (Somatic)
Somatisation - (Somatization)
Sommeil profond - (Torpor)
Somnambulisme - (Sleepwalking)
Somnifère - (Sleeping pill)
Somnolence - (Somnolence)
Son - (Sound)
son - (bran)
Sonde - (Probe)
Soporifique - (Soporific)
Sortie - (Exit)
Sortir - (Leave, to)
Soudain - (Sudden)
Souffle - (blow)
Souffle - (Murmur)

Souffle cardiaque - (Murmur, heart)
Souffrance - (Suffering)
Souffrir - (ill, to be)
Souffrir - (Suffer, to)
Soulagement - (Relief)
Soulagement de la douleur - (Alleviate pain)
Soulager - (Alleviate)
Source - (Source)
Source de la maladie - (Source of the illness)
Sources publiques d'eau - (Public water source)
Sourci - (Eyebrow)
Sourcilière - (Superciliary)
Sourd, sourde - (Deaf)
Sourd-muet - (Deaf-Mute)
Sourire - (Smile)
Sous- alimenté (e - (Malnourished)
Sous- groupe - (Subgroup)
Sous l'effet d'un sédatif - (Sedated)
Sous- mandibulaire - (Submandibular)
Sous- muqueuse - (Submucosa)
Sous- phrénique - (Subphrenic)
Sous-alimentation - (Undernourishment)

Sous-capsulaire - (Subcapsular)
Sous-clinique - (Sub-clinical)
Sous-cotes - (Subcostal)
Sous-cutanée - (Subcutaneous)
Sous-développé (e - (Underdeveloped)
Soya, Soja - (Soy)
Spasme - (Spasm)
Spasme du larynx - (Laryngospasm)
Spasme musculaire tonicoclonique - (Tonic-clonic)
Spasmodique - (Spastic)
Spasticité - (Spasticity)
Spastique - (Spastic)
Spécialiste - (Specialist)
Spécialité médicale - (Medical specialist)
Spécifique - (Specific)
Spectre - (Spectrum)
Spéculum - (Speculum)
Spermatozoïde - (Spermatozoid)
Sperme - (Sperm)
sperme - (semen)
sperme - (sperm)
Spermicide - (Spermicide)
Sphénoïde - (Sphenoid)
Sphincter - (Sphincter)
Sphinctérectomie - (Sphincterectomy)
Spondylite - (Spondylitis)
Sporadique - (Sporadic)
spores - (spore)
Sport - (Sport)
Sprue - (Sprue)
Squelette - (Skeleton)
Staphylococcie - (Staphylococcemia)
Staphylocoque - (Staphylococcus)
Statistique - (Statistic)
Stature - (Stature)
Sténose - (Stenosis)
Sténose mitral - (Mitral valve stenosis)
Stérile - (Sterile)
stérile - (sterile)
Stérilet - (Intrauterine device; IUD)
Stérilisation - (Sterilization)
stériliser - (sterilise)
Stérilité - (Sterility)
Sterno-cléido-mastoïdien,muscle au cou - (Sternocleidomastoid)
Sternum - (Sternum)
Stertor, râle - (Rales; rasping breath)
Stéthoscope - (Stethoscope)
Stigmate - (Stigma)
Stimulant - (Stimulant)
Stimulation - (Stimulation)

Stimulus - (Stimulus)
Stomatite - (Stomatitis)
Strabisme - (Strabismus)
Streptocoque - (Streptococcus)
Streptocoque - (Streptococcus)
Streptokinase - (Streptokinase)
Streptomycine - (Streptomycin)
Stress - (Stress)
Strongyloïdose - (Strongyloidiasis)
Structure - (Structure)
Stupeur - (Stupor)
Style de vie - (Lifestyle)
Suave, doux, douce - (Smooth)
Subaigu - (Sub-acute)
Subdural (le - (Sub-dural)
Subitement - (Sudden)
Subjectif (ive - (Subjective)
Sublingual - (Sublingual)
Subscapulaire - (Subscapular)
Substance - (Substance)
Substitut du lait maternel - (Substitute, breastmilk)
Substitut, remplaçant - (Substitutions; replacement)
Substitution, remplacement

- (Substitution; replacement)
Substrat - (Substrate)
Suc gastrique - (Gastric juice)
Succion - (Suction)
Sucer - (Suck, to)
Sucer - (Suck, to)
Sucre - (Sugar)
Suer, transpirer - (Sweat, to)
Sueur, transpiration - (Sweat)
Sueurs nocturnes - (Sweats, night)
Suffisant (e - (Sufficient)
Suggérer - (Suggest, to)
Suicide - (Suicide)
Suinter, distiller - (Distill)
Suite de couches - (Postpartum period)
Suivant - (Next)
Suivi - (Monitoring (following))
Suivre - (Monitor, to; to follow)
Sulfate de Barium - (Barium Sulfate)
Super infection - (Super-infection)
Superficielle - (Superficial)
Supérieur - (Superior)

Superstition - (Superstition)
Superviser - (Supervise, to)
Supplément - (Supplement)
supplément - (supplement)
Supplément vitaminique -
(Supplement, vitamin)
Suppléments alimentaires -
(Food supplement)
support - (carrier)
Supporter - (Endure, to)
Suppositoire - (Suppository)
Suppression - (Suppression)
Supprimer la lymphe -
(lymph)
Suppuration - (Supperation;
discharge)
Suppurer - (Supperate;
ooze; discharge, to)
Supra claviculaire -
(Supraclavicular)
Supra ventriculaire -
(Supraventricular)
Sûr (e - (Sure)
Sur le dos - (Face up)
Sur le ventre, à plat ventre -
(Face down)
Surdité - (Deafness)
Surdose - (Overdose)
Surpoids - (Overweight)
Surrréflectivité -
(Hyperreflexia)
Survivant - (Survivor)
Survivre - (Survive, to)

Susceptible - (Susceptible)
Suspension - (Suspension)
Suture - (Suture)
suture - (suture)
Suturer - (Suture; stitch, to)
Symétrique - (Symmetric)
Sympathique - (Kind; nice
(a person is...))
Sympatico- mimétique -
(Sympathomimetic)
Symptomatique -
(Symptomatic)
Symptomatologie -
(Symptomatology)
Symptôme - (Symptom)
Symptôme retardé -
(Symptom, late)
Symptômes simulés -
(Symptom, simulated)
Synapse - (Synapse)
Synchronique -
(Syncronous)
Syncope - (Syncope)
Syndrome - (Syndrome)
Syndrome de Down -
(Syndrome, Down)
Syndrome néphrétique -
(Syndrome, nephrotic)
Syndrome respiratoire -
(ARDS)
Synergie - (Synergy)
Synergique - (Synergistic)
Synonyme - (Synonymous)

Synovial - (Synovial)
Synovite - (Sinovitis)
Synthèse - (Synthesis)
Syphilis - (Syphilis)
Syphilitique, luétique - (Syphilitic)
Systématique - (Systematic)
Système de maintien de la vie - (System, life support)
Système de santé - (System, Health)
Systémique - (Systemic)
Systole - (Systole)
Systolique - (Systolic)

~ T ~

Tabac, cigare - (Tobacco)
Tabagisme - (Tobacco poisoning)
Tableau - (Table; Plank)
Tabou - (Taboo)
Tache - (Macule)
Tache - (Stain; blemish)
Tachyarythmie - (Tachyarrhythmia)
Tachycardie - (Tachycardia)
Tachycardie auriculaire - (Atrial flutter)
Tachypnée - (Tachypnea)
Tact - (Touch)

Taille - (Size (as in clothing); waist)
Taille - (Waist)
Talon - (Heel)
Talon d'Achille - (Heel, Achilles)
Tamponnement - (Tamponage)
Tannin - (Tannin)
Tante - (Aunt)
Tard, après midi - (Afternoon; early evening)
Tarse - (Tarsus)
Tartre, saburre - (Tartar)
Taux - (Rate)
Taux d'avortement - (Abortion rate)
Taux de calcium dans l'urine - (Calciuria)
Taux de glucose - (Glucose levels)
Taux de mortalité - (Mortality rate)
Taux de mortalité infantile - (Infant Mortality rate)
Taux de natalité - (Birth rate)
tavelure - (scab)
Technicien de laboratoire - (Laboratory Technician)
Technicien de laboratoire, laborantin - (Lab technician)

Technique - (Technician)
Technologie - (Technology)
Technologie médicale -
(Medical technology)
Teigne - (Tinea)
Télangiectasie -
(Teleangiectasia)
Téléconférence -
(Teleconference)
Tempe - (Temple)
Température -
(Temperature)
Température élevée, fièvre -
(Temperature; fever)
Temps - (Time)
Tendance - (Trend)
Tendinite - (Tendinitis)
Tendon - (Tendon)
tendon - (tendon)
Tendon d'Achille - (Tendon,
Achilles)
Tendu (e - (Tense)
Ténesme - (Tenesmus)
ténia - (tapeworm)
Ténia, ver solitaire - (Tenia)
Ténosynovite -
(Tenosynovitis)
Tension - (Tension;
pressure)
Tension artérielle -
(Pressure, arterial)
Tératogène - (Teratogeny)
Tératogénique -

(Teratogenic)
Tératome - (Teratoma)
Terminal - (Terminal)
Terreur - (Terror)
Test, analyse - (Test; proof;
analysis)
Test, examen - (Test)
Testiculaire - (Testicular)
Testicule - (Testicle)
testicules - (testicles)
Testostérone -
(Testosterone)
Tétanie - (Tetany)
Tétanos - (Tetanus)
Tête - (Head)
Tête - (Head)
Téter - (Suckle, to)
Tétracycline - (Tetracycline)
Tétralogie de Fallot -
(Tetralogy of fallot)
Tétraplégie - (Quadriplegia)
Texture - (Texture)
Thalamus - (Thalamus)
Thalassémie -
(Thalassemia)
Thé - (Tea)
Théophylline -
(Theophylline)
Théorique - (Theoretical)
Thérapeutique -
(Therapeutic)
Thérapie - (Therapy)
Thérapie de

réhydratationorale - (Oral Rehydration Therapy (ORT))
Thermique - (Thermal)
Thermomètre - (Thermometer)
Thermorégulation - (Thermoregulation)
Thiabendazole - (Thiabendazole)
Thiamine - (Thiamin)
Thoracique - (Thoracic)
Thoraco-abdominal - (Thoraco-abdominal)
Thorax - (Thorax; Chest)
Thromboembolie - (Thrombembolism)
Thrombolytique - (Thrombembolytic)
Thrombopénie - (Thrombocytopenia)
Thrombophlébite - (Thrombophlebitis)
Thrombose - (Thrombosis)
Thrombus, caillot sanguin - (Thrombus)
Thymus - (Thymus)
Thyroïde - (Thyroid)
Thyroïdites - (Thyroiditis)
Tibia - (Tibia)
Tibial (le - (Tibial)
Tic - (Tic)
Timbre - (Timbre)

Timolol - (Timolol)
Tique - (Tick)
Tirer - (Throw)
Tirer avec force - (Exacerbation; attack (of disease))
Tissu - (Tissue)
Tissu cutané - (Tissue, subcutaneous)
Tissulaire - (Tissue-like)
Toilettes publiques - (Public bathrooms)
Toiture - (Roof)
Tolérance - (Tolerance)
Tolérance au médicament - (Tolerance to the drug)
Tolérer - (Tolerate)
Tomber malade - (Get sick, to)
Tomographie - (Tomography)
Tomographie Axial par ordinateur (CAT scan - (Computed Tomography (CT))
Tonique - (Tonic)
Tonus - (Tone)
Topique - (Topical; for external use)
Tordu (e - (Sprained)
Torse - (Torso)
Torsion - (Torsion)

Torticolis - (Torticollis)
Total - (Total)
Toucher - (Touch)
Toujours - (Always)
Tousser - (Coughing)
Tout - (All)
Tout petit, minuscule - (Small)
Toux - (Cough)
Toxémie - (Toxemia)
Toxicité - (Toxicity)
Toxicomane - (Drug dependency)
toxicomanie - (Drug addiction)
Toxine - (Toxin)
Toxine tétanique - (Toxin, tetanus)
Toxique - (Toxic)
Toxoïde - (Toxoid)
Toxoplasmose - (Toxoplasmosis)
Trachéal - (Tracheal)
trachée - (Trachea)
Trachéite - (Tracheitis)
Trachéotomie - (Tracheotomy; tracheostomy)
Trachome - (Trachoma)
Tractus - (Tract)
Traduction - (Translation)
Traitement - (Treatment)
Traitement alternatif moins

cher - (Treatment, cheaper alternative)
Traitement ambulatoire - (Treatment, outpatient)
Traitement de l'eau - (Treatment, water)
Traitement de maintient - (Treatment, maintenance)
Traitement préventif - (Treatment, preventive)
Traiter - (Treat)
Tranquille - (Calm)
Tranquille - (Tranquil; calm)
Tranquillisant - (Tranquilizer)
Transaminase - (Transaminase)
Transfert - (Transferral)
Transformer - (Transform)
Transfusion - (Transfusion)
Transfusion sanguine - (Transfusion, blood)
Transitoire - (Transient)
Translocation - (Translocation)
Transmetteur (euse - (Transmitter)
Transmettre - (Transmit)
Transmissible - (Transmissible)
Transmission - (Transmission)
Transpirer - (Perspire;

sweat)

Transplantation, greffe - (Transplant)

Transvaginale - (Transvaginal)

Trauma - (Trauma)

Traumatique - (Traumatic)

Traumatisme - (Traumatism)

Traumatisme obstétricien - (Trauma, Birth)

Travailler - (Work)

Travailleur social - (Social worker)

trèfle - (clover)

Tremblant - (Tremulous)

Tremblement - (Tremor)

Trépanation - (Trepanation)

Tréponème pâle - (Treponema pallidum)

Très - (Very)

Très âgé - (Long-lived)

Triade - (Triad)

Triceps - (Triceps)

Tricyclique - (Tricyclic)

Trigémellaire - (Nerve, trigeminal)

Trimestre - (Trimester)

Triplets - (Triplets)

Trismus, tétanos - (Trismus)

trocart et la canule - (trochar and cannula)

Trois fois par jour - (Three times a day, TID)

Troisième - (Third)

troisième paupière - (third eyelid)

Trompe - (Tube)

Trompe de Fallope - (Tube, fallopian)

Trompe utérine - (Tube, uterine)

Tronc - (Trunk)

Trophique - (Trophic)

Trou - (Hole)

Trouble - (Clouded)

Trouble - (Disorder)

troubler - (Alter)

troubler - (modify)

Troubles mentaux - (Mental disorders)

Trousse à pharmacie, armoire - (Medicine cabinet; medicine kit)

Trousse d'urgence - (First aid kit)

Tube - (Tube)

Tube - (bile duct)

Tubercule - (Tuber)

Tuberculeux - (Tuberculous)

Tuberculine - (Tuberculin)

Tuberculose - (Consumption; Tuberculosis)

Tuberculose - (Tuberculosis)

Tubérosité - (Tuberosity)

Tubulaire - (Tubular)
Tuméfaction - (Swelling)
Tuméfier - (Swell, to)
Tumeur - (Tumor)
Tumeur bénigne/maligne - (Tumor, benign/malignant)
Tumeur de Wilms - (Wilms tumor)
Tumeur primaire - (Tumor, Primary)
Tumeur secondaire - (Tumor, Secondary)
Tumoral (e - (Tumoral)
Turgide - (Tumescent)
twitch - (twitch)
Tympan - (Eardrum; Tympanum)
Tympanite - (Bloat)
Typhoïde - (Typhoid)
Typhus - (Typhus)
Typique - (Typical)

~ U ~

Ulcération - (Ulceration)
Ulcère - (Ulcer, gastric)
ulcère - (ulcer)
Ulcère de décubitus, plaiede lit - (Ulcer, decubitus)
Ulcère peptique - (Ulcer, peptic)
Ulcères - (Ulcers)

Ulcéreux (se - (Ulcerous)
Ultrasonographie - (Ultrasonography)
Une croissance tumorale - (tumour)
Une paralysie - (paralysis)
Uni (e - (United)
UNICEF - (UNICEF)
Unicellulaire - (Single-cell)
Uniforme - (Uniform)
Unilatéral (e - (One-sided; unilateral)
Union - (Union)
Unique - (Unique)
Unir - (Join)
Unités de santé - (Health units)
Universel - (Universal)
Université - (University)
Urée - (Urea)
Urémie - (Uraemia)
Urètre - (Ureter)
Urètre - (Urethra)
Urétrite - (Urethritis)
Urétrite - (Urosepsis)
Urgence - (Emergency)
Urgences - (Emergencies)
Urgent - (Urgent)
Urinaire - (Urinary)
Urine - (Urine)
Urine obscure - (Choluria)
Uriner - (Urinate, to)
uriner - (urinate)

Urique - (Uric)
Urographie - (Urography)
Urologie - (Urology)
Urticaire - (Hives)
Usage - (Use (n.))
User - (Use (v.))
Usure cardiaque - (Cardiac output)
Usure, usage - (Use up)
Utéro- cervical (e - (Uterocervical)
utérus - (uterus)
Utérus - (Uterus; womb)
Uvéite - (Uveitis)
Uvule - (Uvula)

~ V ~

Vaccin - (Vaccine)
vaccin - (vaccine)
Vaccination - (Vaccination)
Vacciné (e - (Vaccinated)
Vagal - (Vagal; vagus nerve, of the)
Vagin - (Vagina)
vagin - (vagina)
Vaginal - (Vaginal)
Vaginite - (Vaginitis)
Vaginose - (Vaginosis)
Vaginose bactérienne - (Vaginosis, bacterial)

Vagolytique - (Vagolytic)
Vagotomie - (Vagotonia)
Vague - (Vagus (nerve); vague; vagrant)
vaisseau lymphatique - (lymph vessel)
Vaisseau sanguin - (Vessel, blood)
Vaisseau-actif - (Vasoactive)
Valeur, courage - (Bravery)
Validité - (Validity)
Valium, diazépam - (Diazepam)
Valve - (Valve)
Valvulaire - (Valvular)
Valvule - (Valve)
Valvule mitrale - (Valve, bicuspid)
Valvule tricuspide - (Valve, tricuspid)
Valvules veineuses - (Valves, venous)
Valvulotomie - (Valvulotomy)
Vaporisateur - (Vaporizer)
Vaporisation - (Vaporization)
Variabilité - (Variability)
Variation - (Variation)
Varicelle - (Chicken Pox)
Varicelle Zona - (Chicken Pox)
Varices - (Varicose veins)

Varicocèle - (Varicocele)
Varié(e - (Varied)
Varier - (Vary, to; change, to)
Variété - (Variety)
Variole - (Small pox)
Variqueux (euse - (Varicose)
Varus - (Bent inward)
Vasculaire - (Vascular)
Vasculite - (Vasculitis)
Vasectomie - (Vasectomy)
Vaseline - (Vaseline)
Vasoconstricteur - (Vasoconstrictor)
Vasoconstriction - (Vasoconstriction)
Vasodilatateur - (Vasodilator)
Vasodilatation - (Vasodilatation)
Vasomoteur - (Vasomotor)
Vasopresseur - (Vasopressor)
Vasospasme - (Angiospasm)
Vecteur - (Vector)
Végétarien - (Vegetarian)
Véhicule - (Vehicle)
Veine - (Vein)
veine - (vein)
Veine ingurgitée - (Vein, engorged)
veines - (Veins)
Veinule - (Venule)

Vénéneux(seuse), venimeux(euse - (Poisonous)
Vénérien - (Venereal)
Vent - (Wind)
Ventilateur - (Ventilator; fan)
Ventilation - (Ventilation)
Ventilation artificielle - (Ventilation, artificial)
Ventouse - (Suction cup)
Ventral - (Ventral)
Ventre - (Belly)
Ventre - (Womb)
Ventriculaire - (Ventricular)
Ventricule - (Ventricle)
Ver - (Worm)
Verbosité - (Verbosity)
Vergeture - (Stria; stretch mark)
Vérité - (Truth)
Vermicide - (Vermicide)
vermiforme - (Vermiform)
Vermisseau - (Vermis)
Verre, vaisseau - (Vessel)
Verrue - (Wart)
Vert - (Green)
Vertèbre - (Vertebrae)
Vertébro-costal - (Vertebrocostal)
Vertex - (Vertex)
Vertige - (Vertigo)
Vertige - (Vertigo; sea

sickness)
Vésicule - (Vesicle; bladder)
Vésicule biliaire - (Gall Bladder)
vésicule biliaire - (gall bladder)
Vessie - (Bladder)
Vessie urinaire - (Urinary bladder)
Veuf/ Veuve - (Widow)
Viande - (Meat)
Vibrion - (Vibrio; vibrion)
Vice - (Vice)
Vide - (Empty)
Vie - (Life)
Vie saine - (Healthy life)
Vieillesse - (Old age)
Vieillir - (Age, to)
Vierge - (Virgin)
Vieux/vieille, personne âgée - (Old man; old woman)
Vigilance - (Observation; vigilance)
Vigilance, surveillance sanitaire - (Surveillance, health)
Villosité - (Villi)
Vin - (Wine)
Violence - (Violence)
Violer - (Rape, to)
Virale - (Viral)
Virémie - (Viremia)

Virilité - (Virile)
Virosite - (Viral illness)
Virulent (e - (Virulent)
Virus - (Virus)
virus - (virus)
Virus de l'immunodéficience Humaine, VIH - (HIV virus)
Visage - (Face)
Visage - (Face)
Viscéral e - (Visceral)
Viscères - (Entrails; innards; bowels)
Viscéromégalie - (Organomegaly)
Viscosité - (Viscosity)
Visible - (Visible)
Vision - (Vision)
Visite - (Visit)
Visite à domicile - (House call)
Visite médicale - (Visit, medical)
Visqueux - (Viscous)
Visuel (le - (Visual)
Vitamine - (Vitamin)
vitamines - (vitamins)
Vitiligo - (Vitiligo)
Vitreux (euse - (Vitreous)
Vivant (e - (Alive)
Voie - (Channel; tract)
Voie orale - (Orally)
Voie rectale - (Rectally)

Voir - (See, to)
Voisin (e - (Neighbor)
Voix - (Voice)
Volonté - (Will)
Volume - (Volume)
Volume sanguin - (Blood volume)
Volumineux - (Bulky; swollen)
Vomer - (Vomer bone)
Vomi, vomissement - (Vomit)
Vomir - (Vomit, to)
Vomissement - (Vomiting, emesis)
Voracité - (Voraciousness)
Vouloir - (Want, to)
Vue - (Vision)
Vue fatiguée - (Eye strain)
Vulnérable - (Vulnerable)
Vulvaire - (Vulvar)
Vulve - (Vulva)
vulve - (vulva)
Vulvite - (Vulvitis)
Vulvo-vaginite - (Vulvo vaginitis)

~ W ~

Warfarine (médicament) mauvaise eau de vie - (Warfarin (a blood thinner medication))
WEB - (Web; internet)

~ X ~

Xanthélasma - (Xanthelasma)
Xanthomatose - (Xanthomatosis)
Xanthome - (Xanthem)
Xanthome - (Xanthema)
Xérodermie - (Xoderma)
Xérophagie - (Xerophagia)
Xérophtalmie - (Xerophthalmia)
Xérostomie - (Xerostomia)
Xiphoïde - (Xiphoid)

~ Y ~

Yoga - (Yoga)
Yogourt - (Yogurt)

~ Z ~

Zéro - (Zero)
Zona - (Zone)
Zona - (Zoster)
Zoonose - (Zoonosis)
zovirax - (Acyclovir)
zovirax - (antiviral)

zygote - (Zygote)